MW01071566

KIATSU

KIATSU
BY KOICHI TOHEI

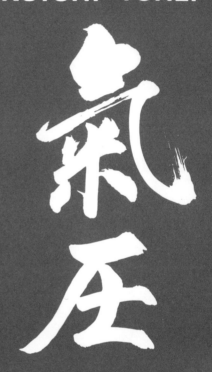

氣圧

KI NO KENKYUKAI H.Q.

© Copyright 1983 by KOICHI TOHEI

All rights reserved. No part of this publication may be reproduced, stored in a retrieval system, or transmitted in any form or by any means, electronic, mechanical, photocopying, recording or otherwise, without the prior written permission of the publisher.

Published by KI NO KENKYUKAI H.Q., Tokyo, Japan.

Distributors:
UNITED STATES: *Kodansha International/USA, Ltd., through Harper & Row, Publishers, Inc., 10 East 53rd Street, New York, N.Y. 10022.* SOUTH AMERICA: *Harper & Row, Publishers, Inc., International Department.* CANADA: *Fitzhenry & Whiteside Ltd., 150 Lesmill Road, Don Mills, Ontario M3B 2T6, Mexico 4, D. F.* BRITISH ISLES: *International Book Distributors Ltd., 66 Wood Lane End, Hemel Hempstead, Herts HPZ 4RG.* EUROPEAN CONTINENT: *Boxer books, Inc., Limmatstrasse 111, 8031 Zurich.* AUSTRALIA AND NEW ZEALAND: *Book Wise (Australia) Pty, Ltd., 101 Argus Street, Cheltenham, Victoria 3192.* THE FAR EAST AND JAPAN: *Japan Publication Trading Co., Ltd., 1–2–1, Sarugaku-cho, Chiyoda-ku. Tokyo 101.*

First edition: June 1983

ISBN 0-87040-536-5

Printed in JAPAN

PREFACE

Why we need Kiatsu Ryoho.

Kiatsu Ryoho is a method to promote human health, encouraging the original life power by sending the Ki of the universe to the damaged part of the body of the patient through the unified body of the healer. Kiatsu means "press with Ki" and Ryoho means therapy.

In ancient Japan it was said that life's span was 50 years and to live seventy years was rare. However nowadays the average life expectancy is 73 for men and 76 for women, thanks to the development of medicine and other advances of civilization.

Most people are dependent on doctors and medication. Many elderly people are spending their lives in bed or in hospitals. To enjoy a long life should mean more than just to stay alive long; one should be able to be healthy all one's life. One of the problems that society now faces is how to make life worth living for retired people, but it would be useless simply to promote leisure activities, when the elderly people are suffering from bodily aches and breathing difficulties. To make life worth living one should be healthy, vigorous, gentle to other people; in sum, one must be needed by others. The key to a life worth living is to be needed by others. Retired people need, above all, to maintain their health. The problem of a society with an ever-growing number of elderly members can also be solved by making young people vigorous and healthy so that one youth can easily earn 5 or 10 retired people's living.

However the reality is that all the nation is half ill and half healthy. It is very rare to find anyone with complete health, while many are dependent on medicine.

In order to solve all these problems I started the "Kiatsu Ryoho School" which I developed through my life-long research. I hope all readers practise so that they can manifest their original Ki power and give it to others. My concern is that as many people as possible should lead a happy healthy life.

CONTENTS

PART TWO : KI EXERCISES FOR HEALTH

PART THREE : MEDICAL LECTURE
(by Dr. Kanemizu Ariizumi)

PART ONE
Kiatsu Ryoho

Chapter $\boxed{1}$ What is Kiatsu Ryoho?

1. Maintenance of health

Everybody wants happiness. The first requirement for happiness is a healthy mind and body. For the mind, please read my "Ki in Daily Life" and "Book of Ki". Here I would like to broach the subject of physical health. To be healthy means to live without physical problems. In other words whether to live a normal life or an abnormal life. Then what is a normal life? Medically speaking life is a metabolism of three things; matter, energy, and form. This is done in the cell body and high metabolism means health, low metabolism means diseases, and when the metabolic process stops, one is dead. Metabolism is the process by which a cell body takes in the nourishment and fuelled by the energy created through the function of enzymes, acts on the substances and finally throwing out the waste materials. In other words we take in the food and water, burn them in our whole body, and change them into energy. This is the physical definition of living. We need oxygen from the air in order to burn the nutriments. Nutrition itself is useless without oxygen. That means breathing is indispensable for living. When the nutriments are burned in the body, naturally carbonic acid gas and other impurities are created. They must be thrown out immediately, otherwise they block the metabolism. Sending the oxygen from the lungs to all parts of the body through the blood stream and taking back the impurities again through the blood stream, the body throws out cabonic acid gas from the nose. This process is vital for the human life.

So the primary requirements for health are good food, good water, and good air. I have been teaching aikido almost every year in Hawaii since 1953. Hawaii is abundant in good food and good water. It has specially good air because it is situated in the middle of the Pacific Ocean. However by no means all the people living on these islands are healthy. There are many people suffering from heart problems, high blood pressure, liver problems, kidney problems, and diabetes. They have as many problems as the Japanese people. It is surprising how many people there are in Hawaii who are suffering from asthma. It is understandable that a place with bad air pollution like Tokyo gives rise to many diseases but it is strange to be ill in a place like Hawaii. The question arises: are food, water, and air in fact sufficient for health? Actually there is one more indispensable thing for the maintenance of health. It is called Ki. Then what is Ki?

2. What is Ki?

In the Japanese language Ki is often used in daily conversation. However even Japanese people have no understanding of Ki. In Japan the source of the absolute universe is traditionally called Ki. Just as the fish forgets the existence of water, the human being also forgets the existence of the Ki of the universe. The reality is that we fix one part of the Ki of the universe with our physical bodies and call it "I". When the human Ki is in interchange with the Ki of the universe, we are alive. When the interchange is temporarily cut off, one faints and if it is cut off eternally, one is dead. We should not forget that we are living in the Ki of the universe.

We more oe less consume Ki while awake. In the morning we are vigorous. By the evening we get tired even if we do nothing in the day time. That is because we consume Ki, just like the battery consumes electricity. We will die if we do not supply Ki after consuming it. Then when do we supply Ki? We do it while asleep. Sleep is a state of complete relaxation when one opens oneself completely to the universe. In this state all the small veins in the whole body are open and the brain is very calm. Just as you can replace dirty air with fresh air by opening the window after using the stove, while asleep the dirty Ki of the human being can be replaced by the Ki of the universe. In the morning we are full of Ki. Perhaps you have not yet fully understood why Ki is indispensable to human life but if you replace the word Ki by the word sleep, it is very easy to understand. Sleep is necessary for human beings. Sleep is the time of repose, the time to renew the supply of Ki, which the universe gives everybody.

Recently many people are irritated, under stress and suffering from nervous ailments. In this way they become rigid, disturbing the blood circulation, and consuming Ki unnecessarily. If you consume too much Ki, you cannot recover completely in one night's sleep. First of all it becomes very difficult to go to sleep. Then many people start depending on sleeping pills. However sleeping pills only create within the body a syncopic state. They do not make the body relax. The cell bodies do not work and there is little interchange between them and the Ki of the universe. In the daytime the Ki is considerably diminished and at night the supply of Ki is cut. Naturally there is not enough Ki. The life power will falter. If you continue living like this, you will surely fall ill and finally die. If you park your car with its lights on, you will find the battery used up. But if you drive it with the lights on, the battery is always automatically charged. We can also charge our bodies with Ki while we are active in the daytime. Then 5 or 6 hours' sleep at night will be enough to be full of Ki. If one extends Ki while awake, one can improve the interchange of the Ki of the human body and Ki of the universe.

3. Life power

Benjamin Franklin said, "A doctor is a person who takes money after God has healed the diseases." Life can be prolonged by the life power. The life power heals the disease and protects our bodies. No doctor nor medicaments can work if there were no life power. The function of the doctor is to discover the disease and think out a method to strengthen the life power. It is the life power which is given by the universe which heals the illness. We take food consciously. But digesting it in the stomach, absorbing the nutriments in the liver and intestines cannot be done consciously. Nor do the nutriments absorbed immediately become our blood and flesh and energy. These nutriments are changed into another form and then changed again into energy. Our bodies are like a very refined chemical factory. The work is done even when we are asleep. What is doing all this work? This question cannot be fully answered even by science or medicine despite their advances. We call it the life power. The universe is one living body. By surrounding a part of it I and my life come in being. Human life cannot be continued independent from the universal life. Oneness with the universe is the essence of human life and when this is achieved the life power can manifest maximum force. If this life power functions strongly all the cell bodies are protected by the life power and work well. Then we can be completely healthy.

Recently many people have forgotten this life power and depend only on doctors and medication. The doctors also tend to forget the life power, relying too much on medication, machines and scientific data. The continual progress of research in the medical field is very important for human beings but such research alone cannot eradicate the causes of illness. All medicine is a help to the life power, though not a substitute for it. In that sense it is a welcomed thing to observe that research in the fields of homeopathic medicine or psychosomatic medicine is gaining recognition world-wide. There are many methods of promoting health but one must be careful to choose the correct methods. A human being cannot exist without following the principles of the universe or nature. The true methods of promoting health must be in accordance with the principles of the universe and nature.

4. How to supply Ki.

When our Ki is interchanging with the Ki of the universe, this creates the most natural and the strongest state with the most vigorous life power. This state is called mind and body unification and by living with mind and body unified, one can stay healthy all through one's life. That is why I am teaching the four basic principles to unify mind and body.

However there are many people who are actually suffering from illness and problems. Once a person has fallen ill or if the body or mind is damaged, one's life power is so low that it is very difficult to recover it by oneself, Sometimes one suffers over 10 or 20 years. In that case we must supply Ki to this person, just as when the power of the battery of a car is drained, it must be charged from outside. By sending Ki into the body from outside, the life power can be encouraged. Once the life power starts working, it can easily heal all illness and problems. This method of sending Ki into the body is named "Kiatsu Ryoho." In order to practise it, one must first know how to extend Ki using the four basic principles to unify mind and body. It is different from Shiatsu, Acupression, Acupuncture, etc., theoretically and practically. If you send your own Ki to others, naturally you consume a lot of Ki. It is no use to fall ill by curing others. One must first learn how to supply Ki from the universe. This is Ki breathing. The Ki of the universe is infinite. If one knows how to supply Ki from the universe, one never lacks Ki however much one sends to others. One must, therefore, know how to unify Ki and how to breathe Ki before learning Kiatsu Ryoho.

Chapter 2 Five Principles of Kiatsu Ryoho

In order to transmit Ki to the body, one must know how to extend Ki and how to send Ki to others. Just imitating the form is no use. One must do everything with correct principles. There are five principles for Kiatsu Ryoho.

1. Extend Ki from the one point in the lower abdomen.

Before sending Ki to others, one must have a body full of Ki and also know how to extend Ki. To keep the one point in the lower abdomen is the first principles of the four basic principles to unify mind and body and one can maintain a body full of Ki by always keeping one point

photo 1

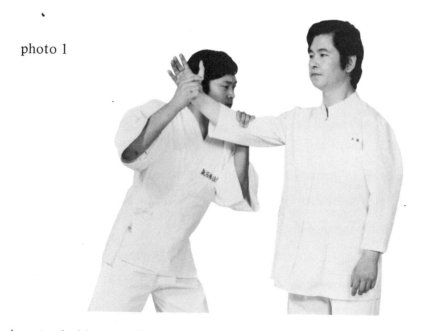

A extends his arm. B tried to bend A's arm by putting his left hand on his elbow and pushing his wrist with the right hand. If A puts strength in his arm and resists, B will be able to bend it easily. If A relaxes and thinks that Ki is flowing through his arm and fingers, B will not be able to bend it however hard he tries. By thinking that Ki is extending one can actually extend Ki.

Arrange the middle three fingers together. B tries to push back the fingertips of A's hand toward the shoulder.

photo 2   photo 3

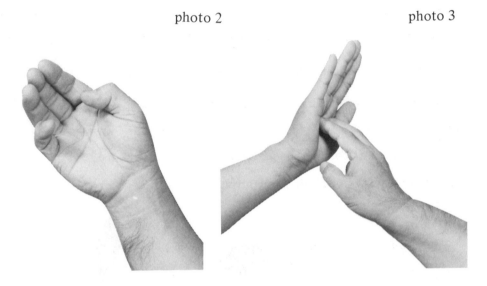

If A puts strength in his fingers or arm, his fingers can easily be bent or pushed back. If A relaxes his arm and fingers and just concentrates on his fingertips which are touching B's palm, B will not be able to bend them. The same thing will happen with the thumb.

When water rushes out from a hose, the highest pressure is at the tip of the hose. In the same way a strong Ki rushing out from the fingers makes the high pressure at the fingertips. In other words focusing sensibility at the fingertips is a method of extending Ki. One must learn to develop this sensibility.

There is also a relation between keeping one point and extending Ki.

All the four basic principles are the same thing expressed differently. If one principle is kept, automatically all the other three are kept. If one principle is lost, automatically all the other three are lost. If one always thinks of extending Ki from the fingertips, one can sometimes fall into an illusion and unconsciously put strength in the arm or shoulders. In that case it is advisable to take the hand off the patient's body, keep one point, and then resume pressing.

(photo 4)

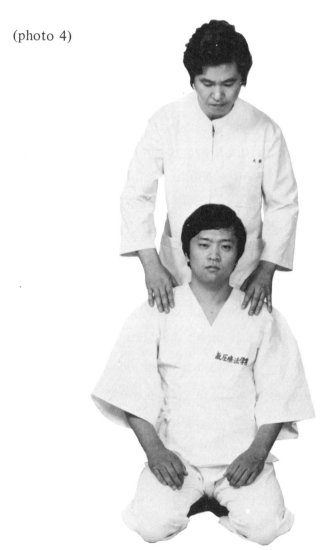

A stands keeping his mind on his one point and extends his arm. He does not have to think Ki is extending. B will not be able to bend the arm.

A stands keeping one point. He does not have to concentrate on his finger-trips. He only puts together his three middle fingers toward B. B tries to push them back with his palm but A's fingers will be very firm. When one point is kept, Ki is naturally extending through the arm and the fingers.

B sits on his knees or cross-legged. A stands behind B and presses with his thumbs on the two points between B's neck and shoulders.   (photo 4)

If A pushes with his thumbs, B will feel pain or an unpleasant sensation of pressure. He will not feel good. But if A presses very lightly, A cannot cure B. Pressing by the power of the thumbs is difficult to regulate and Ki is not extended.

A first keeps one point in the lower abdomen, then puts his thumbs on B's shoulders. First he takes up slack of the soft part under the skin, then he will be able to detect the hard part inside. Do not push farther. Just keep the thumbs there and concentrate Ki on the fingertips. Then the hard place will be gradually softened by the Ki of the fingertips. As it gets softer, the thumbs naturally penerate into B's shoulders. In that case B will not feel much pain. B will be able to feel physically that A's Ki flows into B's body. Sometimes B might feel a little pain on his shoulders but it is a pleasant pain. There is a pleasant pain and an unpleasant pain. Pleasant pain is a sign of healing and unpleasant pain is a sign of getting worse. While doing Kiatsu, sometimes one unconsciously puts strength in the arm or shoulders. Then the Kiatsu is not effective. A gets tired and B has unpleasant pain. A must ask B how he feels. Then there is no mistake. If B feels unpleasant pain or pressure, A should take off his hands and keep one point and then resume pressing.

2. Do not put any strength in the body

To concentrate Ki in the fingertips does not mean to direct strength into the fingertips. If you gather force into the fingertips, the Ki is halted. When the Ki stops, strength accumulates in the arms and other parts of the body. It is useless if you get a stiff shoulder by curing the other's stiff shoulders. If you keep one point and do Kiatsu, it is impossible for strength to gather in your body. However sometimes bad posture or position could cause you to make this mistake.

(photo 5)

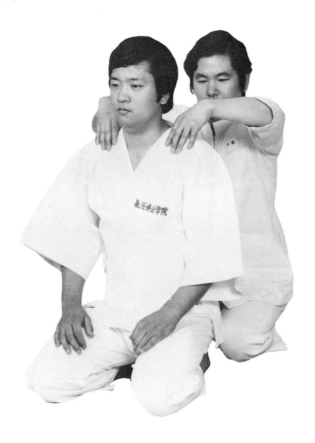

B sits on his knees. A sits behind B and does Kiatsu. A is obliged to keep the arms high in order to press B's shoulders. Even though he tries to relax, strength stays in his arms and shoulders. (photo 5)

B sits with his legs stretched forward. A sits on a chair. Now A's fingers are lower than his shoulders and Ki flows very easily. (photo 6)

B sits on a chair. A stands and does Kiatsu. This position is also easy to extend KI. (photo 7)

(photo 6)

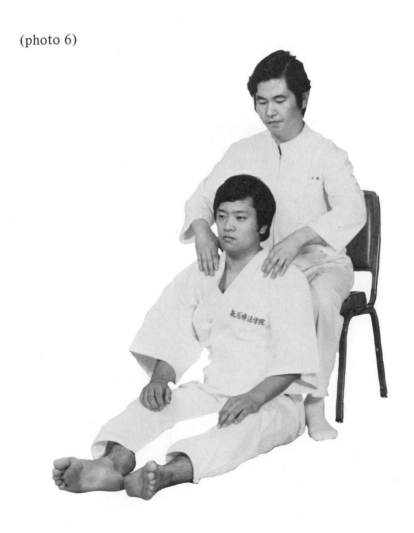

The above examples show that the position relative to the patient is important for relaxation. Always be aware of. this and adopt the easiest posture from which to extend Ki. Sometimes use the middle three fingers instead of the thumbs so that you can extend Ki to the patient without getting tired.

(photo 7)

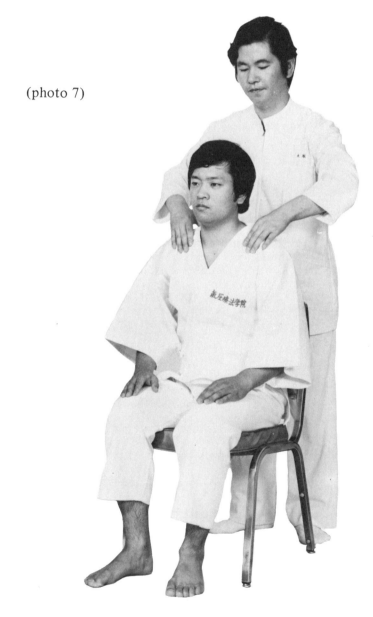

3. Press perpendicularly toward the center without damaging the tissue.

When you pump up a pneumatic tyre, if you put the tip of the air pump into the valve of the tyre correctly, the air goes in easily. But if you place it incorrectly or if you move the tip, the air will not go into the tyre. In the same way when massaging the shoulders, some people try to crumple the

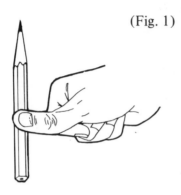

(Fig. 1)

muscles. When the massage is done the muscles become softer and feel good, but it does not last long. Next morning the shoulders become stiffer. As this process is repeated, the muscles and tendons get used to it and lose sensibility. Then however hard they are massaged, they do not feel pain.

If a rubber hose is left outside on a cold winter day for a certain time, it

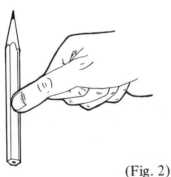

(Fig. 2)

freezes stiff. If one tries to crumple it up, the tissue will be broken. But if one warms it up, it becomes elastic again. In the same way if one tries to crumple the damaged part, the tissue will be broken. The broken tissues will require more energy to recover and so will become stiffer. To that hardened

tissue one should not crumple but just press with the fingertip toward the center of the tendon or muscle perpendicularly and send Ki inside the body. Then the life power will make the tissue soft.

In order to learn how to press perpendicularly to the center, try the following exercise.

A puts a pencil on a table. He presses it with the thumb. B flips the pencil with his forefinger and the middle finger. If A presses the pencil obliquely as in figure 1, the pencil will be flipped away by B easily no matter how A tries to press it. If A puts the thumb perpendicularly to the table and presses the pencil with a relaxed thumb thinking that his Ki penetrates through the pencil to the table, the pencil can move but never leaves A's thumb when flipped by B. In that case the Ki from A's thumb is actually penetrating the pencil.

4. Concentrate Ki infinitely smaller at the fingertips.

The effect of Kiatsu Ryoho differs greatly according to the strength of Ki of the healer. The strength of Ki depends on the concentration of the mind. When I give seminars in the U.S.A. or Europe, I sometimes invite people who have physical problems such as migraine headaches, stiff shoulders, whiplash, sciatic pain, sprain, etc. Five minutes' treatment each and their pain is gone. In five minutes the headache will have vanished, the arm can go up, a person who came limping with a stick can run without a stick. The audience is always surprised. Yet this miracle can be achieved by everybody. The only difference is whether it takes five minutes or several hours. The life power is very great. The secret of Kiatsu Ryoho is to activate the life power. To do this one must practise to extend Ki very strongly with concentration. As you practise, you can shorten the time. In all probability many people will have difficulty understanding what I mean by the instruction to concentrate Ki infinitely smaller at the fingertip. Nowadays science has developed an atomic bomb which is small enough to put in a bag, yet when exploded wipes away a whole town. The smaller the particle is, the stronger energy it can generate. The same is true of the mind. The more it is concentrated, the stronger its power becomes. This is Ki meditation.

Mathematically speaking, first assume one. Half of one also becomes one. If one is divided by half infinitely, it is always one and never becomes zero. Zero can never produce one. The universe is an assembly of infinitely small particles. These constitute the Ki of the universe. The absolute quantity of the Ki of the universe does not change. It does not increase or decrease. But it is a transmutable continuum flowing without a break as time does. The universe itself is an infinite circle of an infinite radius. I am the center of the universe because wherever I am, the universe is always infinite in all directions. When one understands the nature of the universe, one can be one with the universe.

Try to think while sitting calmly. The universe is an infinite circle with an infinite radius. This universe condensed becomes myself and again condensed becomes my one point in the lower abdomen. This one point is not a tangible point but an infinitely small point which keeps on getting smaller. When the one point is too small to perceive, just let it continue. Do not stop its movement. This is Ki mediatation.

By thinking like this you can become one with the essence of the universe. You will be very stable mentally and physically. This is called keeping one point in the lower abdomen. In this state a very strong Ki flows out of the fingertips naturally. However when the patient has a very grave problem, the stiff part does not yield easily. If you take time and apply Kiatsu many times you will succeed in making it soft but if you want to achieve the result more quickly, you can use this method of concentrating Ki infinitely smaller at the fingertip. The fingertip is a round circle. This circle is one. Make it half. Even though it becomes infinitely smaller by half, you must continue making it smaller. (figure 3)

In this way a very strong Ki will flow out of the fingertip which will make the stiff part soft. The fingertip will be very sensitive so that you can detect the new line which you did not find before. A beginner should practise this method, gaining the awareness of the infite concentration of Ki at the fingertips at every opportunity. He will surely progress in Kiatsu Ryoho and in the Ki power.

(Fig. 3)

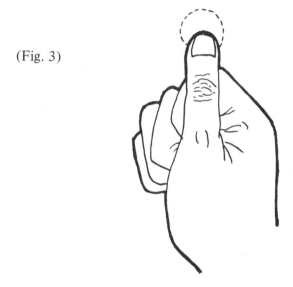

5. Think of the lines instead of points.

When you travel along a highway, you pass many interchanges. But you do not have to know all the interchanges. By following the highway you can naturally reach the destination. Similarly there are many points in the human body. They are like interchanges. Many nerves converge on and diverge from those points. It is very difficult to learn all the points of the body because the position of each point changes according to the posture of the body. However the human body is a unified entity. All the nerves connect to form various flows between the brain and the whole body. By following all the line, one can easily pass all the points just as you can pass all the interchanges by travelling down the highway. That is why I do not teach points but only lines. One can do Kiatsu at all the parts of the body. It does not take much time to learn the important lines. Instead of taking a great deal of time to learn the points, it would be better to learn how to extend Ki.

Chapter $\boxed{3}$ How Kiatsu Ryoho Was Developed

People have heard of massage, shiatsu, acupuncture, acupression, moxa-cuatery, etc. But few people have heard of the name "Kiatsu Ryoho". This is because I personally developed Kiatsu Ryoho and I have not until now tried to introduce it to the world.

However in the world nowadays people have become aware of the danger of taking medicaments. That is why I established a school of Kiatsu Ryoho to teach it and to send the pupils to the world in their turn so that they can cure and help the people who are suffering from ailments of mind and body. This method was thus named "Kiatsu Ryoho" because it uses the Ki of the universe sending it to the body and stimulating the original life power which is given by the universe. I have never learned it from anybody. Of course I got several ideas from my training in many disciplines but my teacher was the universe itself. When I ask the universe to teach me, the universe teaches me. In this universe there has always been Ki and the Ki principles. People only do not notice it. I just happened to open my eyes to them.

When I was small I was very weak. My father, who was a fourth dan at judo and very strong, wanted to make me strong. He made me practise judo. Gradually I became stronger. When I entered university, I enlisted in the judo club. However in the spring training camp, I hit my chest during practice. Every evening my chest started to pain me. I went to the hospital and they immediately diagnosed pleurisy and put me in hospital. I wasted one year of university constantly in and out of the hospital. Both my mind and body which had been somewhat strengthened by judo became again very weak. While convalescing, I was much in frustration. "My mind and body

are so weak. What should I do with myself? Will I be like this for the life?"
My home in the country was the old family house and there are many books
in the library. I started reading them. There were many classics from China, a
bible and biographical literature of the world. While I was reading them, I
felt very good but after reading them I was still myself, easily frustrated or
irritated; a weak boy. I then began to realize that it is no use just reading
books and understanding them in head alone. I needed an approach that involved both my mind and body.

After resuming my study in the university, I had an opportunity to
enter the Ichikukai which was led by Master Tetsuju Ogura who was a
student of Yamaoka Tessu. I practised misogi there and also zen with
Master Josei Ota. I practised all day without studying the school subjects of
the university. During this period I vaguely realized that the absolute universe is called Ki and we are one with the universe.

In 1942, 27 September I graduated from Keio University six months early
due to the war, entered the army school, and was sent to China. I spent two
years and half in China until 1945. After the war I again devoted myself to
training, drawing on the experiences I had had in the battle field. In 1953 I
went to Hawaii to spread aikido. Since then I have been conducting seminars in more than twenty states of the U.S.A. and in Europe. I have taught
many big men who are twice as big as I am. If I had relied on physical
strength alone, it would have been impossible to do this. I fortunately learned the Ki principles and knew principles of mind and principles of body
which made it possible. As a result of my training and experience I had
absolute confidence in the existence of Ki. I naturally grasped Kiatsu Ryoho.

Our Ki is one part of the Ki of the universe and life means interchange of
our Ki with the Ki of the universe. Health means to leave oneself open to
the movement of the universe and become one with the universe. In this

instant the life power manifests its maximum force. When the interchange with the universe is disturbed, one gets unhealthy.

For example when the blood circulation is normal, there is no possibility of illness. If the blood circulation is disturbed, many ailments occur. In restoring the blood circulation to normal, the life power is activated and naturally cures the illness. When the interchange with the Ki of the universe is disturbed, Ki is lacking in the body. Kiatsu is to send Ki into the body to supply the shortage and restore the Ki so that the life power is once again activated.

Throughout my life I have been making efforts to understand the Ki of the universe. In response the universe gave this Kiatsu Ryoho to me. I would like to teach this to as many as people as possible. Those who have grasped the principles of the universe have a duty to teach them to others. The experiences of a lifetime have made me realize that Kiatsu Ryoho is a fascinating study. I will give you several examples from my experiences.

1. Diarrhoea in the battle field

In 1944 February I was sent to China and marched from Nanking to Hankow. It is much easier to sail up the Yantze River or to go by train, but in that period the Americans had command of the air in China and using ship or train would have meant instant death at the hands of the American air force. After several days' march, we took a rest in a small town. I bought a meat bun in a small shop. At night I had an acute stomachache. The meat in the bun must have been bad. The medicine did not work at all. There was no doctor at hand. Having no other resources I pressed my belly with my fingertips. In the Japanese language to cure is "teate o suru" (put a hand on). I thought that by sending Ki with my hand I could ease the pain. After a while the pressing eased the pain, then suddenly I wanted to go to toilet.

There was a violent purging. The pain subsided. Then in less than five minutes the pain returned. I again pressed with my fingers and then again relief came through purging. 17 times in that night I repeated the treatment. At around two o'clock in the morning the pain was completely gone and I could sleep well. Next morning I started marching without breakfast. By noon I was hungry. I ate lunch and my stomach was completely all right. It was my first experience of the effect of extending Ki from the fingertips. After that experience every time my soldiers had diarrhoea, I cured them in the same way. I had 80 soldiers in my troop, but nobody died or fell seriously ill during two and a half years in the Chinese battle field. I think it was partly due to the power of Ki.

2. Curing eye disease.

The war ended. But we had to stay in China for nearly one year before we could go back to Japan. One morning when I awoke, I could not open my eyes because of a sticky secretion collecting in the eyes. I washed my eyes with hot water and could open them but the eyes were sticky and there were small particles behind the eyelids. I went to junior high school by bicycle when I was small. My eyes were always exposed to the cold wind during the winter. In that period my eyes suffered from the wind and in the early spring I always had trachoma. After one or two months' treatment at the hospital, it was all right but next spring again the same thing would happen. So I always carried medicine for my eyes. When I started for the war, I carried a lot of medicine but I lost most of it on my travels. By the time the war had finished I had run out of the medicine. I did not know when we would be allowed to go back to Japan. There was no hope of having medicine sent from Japan. I was at a loss to know what to do with my eyes. So I washed my hands well and put my fingertips on the eyelids where I felt small particles inside. After ten minutes or so the small particles were gone. I changed the position of my fingertips. I continued in this way until there were no small particles behind the eyelids. Then I put clean water in a ball and washed my eyes with the water. Then my eyes were very clear. The small particles behind the eyelids were all washed away. Then I put my three middle fingers on the eyelash. There was a little pain. After a while the pain was gone. Next morning there was only half the sticky secretion as there had been. On the third day there was hardly any secretion. I continued Kiatsu for a week and since then I have never had problems. It is already more than thirty years since then and I have never been to an eye doctor. Sometimes when I did not sleep enough or was too much tired, I felt a bit strange at my eyes. Then I always put my fingers on them and cured them immediately.

3. Giving the name of Kiatsu.

In August 1946 we were finally allowed to return to Japan. I started farming at home in the country and resumed misogi training at Ichikukai dojo and also went to Master Morihei Ueshiba who was also farming in another part of the country. In that quiet country life, I reflected on the busy army life, on how the people behaved on the borderline between life and death, misery of people in the face of death. There were many reflections but all of them were valuable teachings. Also now I knew from experience the difference between the real fighting in the war and the daily aikido practice in the dojo. It was likewise the experience of the battle field which taught me that putting strength in the lower abdomen is wrong. First of all marching is impossible if one puts strength in the lower abdomen. The lower abdomen is a place to calm the mind, not a place to put physical strength.

When I remembered the diarrhoea and my eyes, I did not know whether I had been able to cure them because of the special situation on the battle field or if I could do the same in normal situations. I tried pressing with my fingers when the children had stomachache or the elderly people had neurgia. I found I could cure them in the same way. I thought on this seriously and hit upon the idea of Ki which I had vaguely felt during my training in zen and misogi. Life means the continual interchange of the Ki of the universe and personal Ki. When the interchange is weak and there is a shortage of Ki, one falls ill. If there is a shortage of Ki, supplying Ki can activate the interchange. Pressing with Ki means to give Ki to the damaged part and activate the life power. It is same as charging a weak battery. Everybody can do it if he knows how to extend Ki. The ancient people may well have known it because they did not have any medicine. That might be why there is a Japanese expression "teate o suru" (put a hand on). On realizing it I named my method Kiatsu, meaning pressing with Ki.

4. A blister on the foot.

It was when I went to train in aikido under Master Morihei Ueshiba. I helped him in the fields wearing a pair of shoes which happened to be there. When I finished work I found a big blister on my foot. It was very painful and I had difficulty putting on my own shoes. I put my fingers on it while talking with others. After a while there was no more pain. The blister had broken. I put on my stockings and shoes. The pain was completely gone.

5. Heart problem   (1)

One day a man in his thirties came to see me. He had a pain in the heart and doctor's medicine and injections had no effect. At first I refused, saying I was not a doctor, but he insisted. I told him to lie down on his back and put my hand on his heart. The heart was beating very rapidly and he had difficulty in breathing. His whole body was bloated. I did Kiatsu at his chest and belly. After that his breathing became much easier. After a few days he was much better and I suggested him to see the doctor again. The doctor was puzzled. The beating had become normal. Technically it is impossible for the heart to recover so quickly. However, this time, the doctor who had had experience of the battle field noticed something and gave the patient a medicine for expelling worms. More than a hundred worms were expelled. The cause of the heart problem was the worms, but as the doctor was worried about the heart, he did not notice the worms. Kiatsu made the worms gradually go down to the stomach and the doctor could judge the symptoms correctly.

6. My father's sciatica.

Once while cleaning the house my father tried to lift something heavy and sprained his loin. He could not so much as straighten his body and had to walk with a walking stick even in the house. By that time I had a reputation as a healer and there were many people from the village and the neighbouring villages who came to see me. However my father was doubtful about it and though I suggested that I could cure him, he went to see a doctor. He received many injections but did not recover at all. Then he went for massage, shiatsu, electric treatment, acupuncture, etc. His condition did not improve. After a month he finally gave up and asked me if I could really cure him. I said I could, but added that unless he kept quiet and promised not to tell me what to do while I was treating him, I would not be able to cure him. He answered that he would keep silent and do what I told him. It must have been really galling for him. My father who was usually very stubborn and arrogant was going to have to listen to me. I did Kiatsu in the morning and evening and by the third day there was no pain. But all he said was "I feel a bit better." However after a while when his friend came to visit him he said, without knowing that I was in the next room listening, "It was very magical. I did not believe it at first but my son completely cured my sciatica while everyone else failed."

7. Arm problem.

In February 1953 I left Japan for Hawaii in order to spread the practice of aikido. I opened two places in Honolulu and taught many people every evening. After the evening class I would return to the hotel and spend the night by myself. Later my students invited me to dinner after practice and I had no spare time but at first I was left alone in the hotel. My travel was sponsored by the Hawaii Nishi Association. The Nishi Association is teaching a method to promote health. Dr. Kurisaki who was a vice president of the Nishi Association and president of the judo association of Hawaii as well as a dentist, took good care of me and later became the first president of the Hawaii Aikikai. One evening after class he came to invite me to go out to a ballroom dancing school in Waikiki. His friend, Mr. Hamasaki was teaching dance there. He was very strict on rhythm and danced very well, combining a deep knowledge of music with perfect harmony. I noticed however that his right hand was moving a bit lamely. After the lesson Dr. Kurisaki came to ask me to cure Mr. Hamasaki's right arm. He told me that when Mr. Hamasaki was dancing in a hotel, he fell over on a bad dance floor and hurt his right arm, so that now he could not lift it. That was the reason of the lame movement. Dr. Kurisaki took me there because I had cured his hand when he injured it a few days before. I did Kiatsu on Mr. Hamasaki's arm. Soon he could stretch his arm straight up and could swing freely without pain. Everyone was surprised. This incident gave me the chance to learn ballroom dancing. We were good friends for more than twenty years until Mr. Hamasaki died of old age.

8. Nose bleed.

In May 1953 the All Judo Championship was held in California. Even Canada and Mexico sent participants. Dr. Kurisaki took four participants to the tournament. I was also invited to demonstrate aikido to the assembled judo players. The tournament lasted for two days and on the second day I had five judo players attack me at the same time. I threw them twenty or thirty times in the big dojo. This incident made the name of aikido well-known to judo players in U.S.A. It was a memorable occasion for me, too. Before my demonstration there were the finals of the junior class. One boy was very good and were through to the finals. During the final game his opponent's hand hit the nose of the boy which started bleeding. He could not continue the game. He started crying. I talked to Dr. Kurisaki and stopped the game. Then I went to the boy and had him sit down with a towel on his nose. I supported his head with my left hand and lightly hit his neck with my right hand giving a shout of, "Iei". The bleeding stopped immediately. Much to the boy's surprise I told him to continue the game. They resumed the game which the boy went on to win and so take the championship. The audience clapped enthusiastically for a long time.

9. Migraine headache (1)

In June 1953 I returned from California to Hilo, Hawaii. I was staying in a small hotel run by a Japanese. The Japanese woman who was managing the hotel was in her fifties and suffered from rightly attacks of migraine. Once the pain started at night it would last for several hours. She had to take medicine to prevent the pain. Initially she took one pill every evening but as her resistance to the medcine grew she had to increase the dose so that in those days she had to take two pills. The pills were so strong that they were affecting her health. The hair at the top of her head had become white. She asked me if I could help her. She had heard from her friends in Honololu that I had cured many people. I replied, "It can be cured. Tonight go to bed without taking the medicine. If you had a headache in the night, wake me up." In the evening I did Kiatsu on her head, neck, and shoulders. That night she did not come to wake me. The next morning she said she had been able to sleep very well and she felt fine. When she was taking the medicine she did not feel well in the morning. While staying in that hotel I did Kiatsu on her every evening. After one week or so, I was invited to dinner late in the evening. I telephoned to the hotel to say that I would stay away for the night. That night at around 11 o'clock there was a phone call from the woman who asked me to go back immediately for she had a headache. I was doubtful but went back to make sure. By the time I reached the hotel she was already fine. She was only afraid that the headache might start once she was left alone. I explained her how the mind affects the body. She had never had a headache again. After she stopped taking the medicine for a year her hair all became black again. The white hair was due to the medicine.

10. Knees and arms

In August 1953 I moved to Maui Island. I stayed on Honolulu for six months but on each of the other islands I stayed only one and a half months. It is not easy to teach aikido in one and a half months and educate instructors who had to continue the dojo later. I first had to choose good instructors. Then I gave an instructor's training every morning from 6 to 7 o'clock. The instructor of Maui was Mr. Suzuki of the Maui police. He came to Japan to train and later became the chief instructor of the Hawaii Ki Society. I gave morning and afternoon class to all the police in Maui. Mr. Suzuki was taking care of me all the time during that one month by the order of the chief of police. In the morning at six he and I practiced together. Mr. Suzuki was nearly six feet tall but had not trained as much as I. In fifteen minutes he was already tired. I was young and my technique was still rough. Mr. Suzuki hurt his knees. Next day he said he could not practice because of the knees so I did Kiatsu on them. Then we started practice. After a few days he hurt his arm. I cured it with Kiatsu. We never missed practice. "Tohei sensei, Can Kiatsu be done only by you?" "No, everyone can do it if he knows how to extend Ki." "Then could you please teach me?" I taught him Kiatsu specially. Later he helped the mayor of Maui, the chief of police, and others.

11. Neuraglia of the Arm

In September 1953 I again travelled to Kauai island. Because I gave classes to all the policemen of Maui, chief of the police in Kauai gave an order for all his men to learn aikido from me. During that month a Mr. Uchida was taking care of me. One day I was invited to a student's house. I found his grandmother massaging her shoulders and arms. I asked her what was the matter. She said she had had neuralgia for three months and nothing could cure it. I did Kiatsu for thirty minutes. After that she had no pain.

12. Migraine Headache (2)

In Kauai a man in his thirties came to see me. The upper left part of his face was burned. He explained that the upper left part of his face became very painful around 5 o'clock every afternoon. Nothing could help it. But after one or two hours the pain always went away. When it got painful he put a hot towel on his face to ease the pain. That was why his face was burned. The doctors in Kauai could not help him so he went to Honolulu, but no one knew what to do. In one hospital of Honolulu they suggested cutting one tendon of his face. He asked if cutting the tendeon would stop the pain. The doctors said since it was their first time to see such a case, they could not tell until they tried. He could not decide whether to get operated or not so he came back to Kauai and happened to hear about me. It was the first case of this kind for me too. I touched his face and neck and found a big hard lump around the seventh vertebra. The messages from the brain pass down the spinal column and reach all over the body. An obstacle in the spinal column will disturb the whole function of the body. I decided first to get rid of this obstacle. I first did Kiatsu on his neck and shoulders and then sent Ki to the lump. After a while the hard part got softer. I sent him back at only this state the first day, but he did not have pain that afternoon. He was happy and I was also encouraged, for I had found the cause of the headache. After one week or so the hard part became soft as it should be. Since then he has never had pain and he lives happily and enjoys fishing.

13.　Stomache

In October 1953 I went back to Honolulu after Hawaii, Maui, and Kauai. One day during the practice a Mr. Inoue suddenly developed a severe stomach-ache. He bent over clutching the pain. I stopped class and did Kiatsu on his stomach. After about ten minutes he got up saying that the pain had subsided and resumed practice. All the other aikidoists were surprised. Later Mr. Inoue and others came to ask me to teach them Kiatsu Ryoho. I said I would teach those who would teach others aikido even after I went back to Japan. This news went to the other islands and I had to again visit the other three island for 15 days each to teach Kiatsu.

14. Stiff Neck

In 1955 I went to Hawaii for the second tme. When I arrived at Maui, Mr. Suzuki came to meet me at the airport and took me immediately to the Maui Hospital. He took me to the doctor's room. The doctor was scheduled to do an important operation that afternoon. But in the morning when he woke up, he had a stiff neck and could not even move the head. The other doctors tried to help him without success. A stiff neck will naturally go away in a week or so but in that case he had to be ready for the operation that afternoon. The head nurse heard about that and said her husband might be able to do something. Her husband was Mr. Suzuki. Mr. Suzuki received a telephone call from his wife but did not have enough confidence to cure it immediately. Luckily I was due to arrive that morning. That was why he was waiting for me. I immediately applied Kiatsu. First I made the neck soft and then bent it well in all directions. When the tendons and muscles became soft and elastic, it did not hurt. After thrity minutes of Kiatsu I told him to move as he wanted. The doctor swung his head and arms and tried all possible movements. The pain was completely gone. Other doctors were all astonished. The   operation was successful. Later Mr. Suzuki was often asked to cure such cases at the hospital.

15. Sprained Ankle

In April, 1956, after coming back from my second trip to the U.S.A., I was asked to be the director and the chief instructor of Aikikai. My master, Morihei Ueshiba, was teaching in another part of Japan and he asked me to come immediately. So I took a night train from Tokyo. In the morning a man in his thirties starting for the toilet sprained his ankle. He was complaining that his ankle hurt too much for him to walk with his two big trunks. I woke up and did Kiatsu for fifteen minutes. He could then move his foot freely. I asked him to walk. He first hesitated but found there was no pain and started for the toilet. A young student who was accompanying me got angry saying that the man did not know very good manners for he went away without thanking me. I said it was all right. He probably forgot to thank me because he was so surprised that he could walk so easily. I was right. After coming back from the toilet, the man came and thanked me very politely.

16. Stroke

In September, 1957, during my third trip to Hawaii, I was practicing on Hawaii island. I received news that Mr. Tutsui of Oahu island had a stroke of apoplexy. He was nearly 60 years old and taking care of judo and sumo in the Wailuku area. He also had taken good care of me. In October when I went to Oahu, he was recuperating at home. He was very happy to see me but the left side of the body was paralysed. However, he could move his left hand for ten centimeters or so and he could move his left knee a little. That was a proof that the muscles were not dead yet. I tried Kiatsu on him and each time he could move his body better. I went to do Kiatsu several times and then he could speak much more clearly. After three years Mr. and Mrs. Tutsui came to see Japan and told me that he could walk up the Tokyo tower. He recovered so that he could live his daily life almost normally.

17. Eye Problems

In 1958 after my third trip to the U.S.A. Mr. Inoue was trying to clean a room with a disinfectant. He mishandled the apparatus and got the disinfectant in his eyes. He had a terrible pain and was taken to hospital but the doctors said his eye sight was lost. All the other doctors were in the same opinion. He was very discouraged, but a few days later he remembered Kiatsu and thought, "If I am already blind, my eyes cannot be worse than now." He did Kiatsu on his eyes all day long since he had nothing else to do. Then gradually his paralysed eyes regained sense and he could feel pain. Then he started to feel the light. Encouraged he continued Kiatsu and at last recovered his eyesight. He immediately wrote me a letter of thanks. He can drive a car and continues practice even now.

18. Heart Problem

In 1960 I received a letter from Hawaii saying that Mr. Eto was sent to the hopistal with serious heart problem. Mr. Eto was an architect and had been practising since 1953, my first trip to Hawaii. Later he went to Guam for his work and in several years established the Guam Aikikai. In Guam it is very hot and humid, so one easily perspires. He was taking a salt pill after practice. I, too, was advised by someone in Hawaii to take salt pills but I stopped immediately for I found the salt pill was not good for me. But Mr. Eto was taking two salt pills every day. That was why he was hospitalized after coming back to Hawaii for heart problem. Salt is necessary but too much salt is not good. I immediately replied to him, "There is nothing you can do in the hospital. While lying in bed, put your hand on your heart and send Ki to it. Practise breathing methods well. Do not do a long breathing at first. First keep one point and breathe out as calmly as possible and wait a second and breathe in from the nose. After breathing in, wait a few seconds and then breathe out. Continue this and you will be able to breathe very easily and deeply. Then your life power will be considerably activated." Mr. Eto knew breathing methods but he preferred to practice aikido techniques and did not practise breathing very much. After my letter he faithfully practised correct breathing. He recovered very rapidly and soon left the hospital. Now, in 1982 he is 75 years old and still one of the best instructors in the Hawaii Ki Society, teaching Ki and aikido vigorously besides managing his own business. He always continues breathing and says that he could live happily thanks to my teachings.

19. The Backbone

In February, 1961, on my fourth trip to Hawaii, I took master Morihei Ueshiba to Hawaii. At that time aikido had already spread all over Hawaii and most policemen in Hawaii took aikido lessons. The chief and vice-chief of police of Honolulu were taking private lessons with me. I was bestowed the title of honorary captain of the Honolulu police and the Maui police. All Hawaii welcomed my master. When master, my students, and I went in a car caravan, policemen on motorcycles escorted us in front and back. We continued without regard to the traffic lights while all the other cars waited. It was only the President of the U.S.A. who received this VIP treatment. From Japan only the prince was received like this. Mr. Inoue, who recovered his eyesight, was very well at that time but said, "My wife has a numb leg. I took her to hospital and the doctor said the backbone requires an operation. I knew you were coming so I waited for your opinion," I said, "The operation is the last thing to do. Once your body is operated upon, it will never be the same. If it is an acute disease, sometimes an operation is necessary but only a numb leg can wait. Do what you can do, and if everything fails, then have the operation. You recovered from blind. Why don't you do Kiatsu on her spine?" "The doctor prohibited me from toching her spine." "When he wants to go so far as to cut it, why should it not be touched? Kiatsu is only to touch and send Ki. It will never make it worse. If your Kiatsu does not work, I will do it. If I cannot cure it, then operate." Mr. Inoue did Kiatsu on the lines beside the spine and after a few days there was a faint sound. After that the leg regained feeling. It was cured. The vertebra must have slipped out of the place and suppressed the nerve. The muscles and tendons were fixed arount it, but when he was doing Kiatsu the muscles and tendons relaxed and the bone must have come into the correct position again. She did not have any problems since then.

20. Stiff Shoulders

After Master Ueshiba stayed in Hawaii for one and one-half months in 1961 he went back home. I went around the Hawaiian Islands and then for the first time went over to the continental United States to spread aikido. My students in Hawaii went to Los Angeles and San Diego and started Aikikai dojos there. This time they invited me for seminars. In Los Angeles a student brought his sister. She had very stiff shoulders. Naturally she also had a headache. She had her shoulders massaged every day but at that time massage had no effect on her shoulders. I touched her shoulders and found that the surface was not so hard but the inside was hard. Normally when I did Kiatsu both the patient and I could feel that my Ki goes into the body. But in her case it was like pressing on rubber and my Ki did not penetrate. I asked her how she made her shoulders like they were. She said, "Before, my shoulders were not like this. I liked being massaged so whenever I felt stiff I had my shoulders massaged. Immediately after massage I felt well but the next morning my shoulders were always stiffer. So I had massage again. Repeating this made my shoulders very stiff." In Japan we call it, "The shoulders which kill the masseur". However hard one kneads she does not feel pain. She asks to knead harder and the masseur gets tired out. Hence they are the shoulders which kill the masseur. Stiff shoulders are also a disease. If one tries to knead them in order to soften them, it breaks the tissues. This is why in the next morning the shoulders get stiffer. Repeating this process makes the shoulders hard and rubbery. It is no use to knead. I put my thumbs on the points between the neck and the shoulders and pressed a little and stayed there calmly. "I do not feel anything." "Be silent. I have started." As I concentrated my Ki on the thumbs by halves, my Ki started to penetrate into her body little by little. In a few minutes my Ki went through her muscle and reached at the hard core. When my fingertip touched the hard muscles there, she cried of pain. After that it was much easier. I could easily touch the other part of the hard core. She was crying in pain all the time. In fifteen minutes she felt that her shoulders were so light. She asked me, "So I will not have any more stiff shoulders?" "Yes, you will have stiff shoulders again." "Then you did not cure them completely." "Yes, I cured them. But think a little. When you were a baby, you did not have any stiff shoulders. Your shoulders became stiff after you became adult. That means your mistakes in your daily life made the shoulders stiff. If you repeat the same mistakes your shoulders will again be stiff." She told me she typed all day long. In the morning she was relaxed but in the afternoon she tensed because of fatigue. The same problem applied to pianists and barbers. So I taught her to keep one point and relax completely and also taught Ki exercises which prevent stiff shoulders. Later she did not have stiff shoulders and could type much better than before.

21. Stomach Ulcer

In 1968when I was teaching in New York for four months, I had already established Aikikai dojos in Calfornia, Illinois, Wisconsin, Pennsylvania, Ohio, and Georgia. On the East Coast I had dojos in New York and Chicago. When I was young I was a heavy drinker and had a reputation for that. The instructor of New York, Mr. Yamada, suggested me to drink a cocktail instead of whisky and soda before dinner. I tried the cocktail and found it very tasty. After the evening class I drank cocktails and forgot to have dinner. The cocktail was strong and contained heavy liquor. After this I drank whisky and soda till late at night. In four months I damaged my stomach. After New York I taught in Chicago for two months and San Francisco for one month. Though my stomach was not good, I was still drinking beer. In October when I went back to Los Angeles I could not sleep one night because of the pain in the stomach. The next day and the day after I had blood in my feces. I went to Dr. Omori who was my student. Dr. Omori immediately took me to a big hospital and took 30 or 40 X-ray photos. The next day I went to see him again and he told me there was one big ulcer and two small ulcers. There was nothing wrong with my liver and kidneys. The doctor suggested operating immediately but I refused. He said, "I can wait for one month. After one month if the ulcer gets worse, let me operate." I said, "All right. If it gets better after a month, then I do not need an operation." He agreed, "If it gets better , an operation is unnecessary." I announced that I would be better. In Los Angeles I had to teach for two months. The doctor suggested me to be quiet but I never stopped teaching. So my students did not know I had an ulcer. Naturally I stopped drinking and did not eat sweet or salty things. I had already stopped smoking. I did Kiatsu for one hour each morning and evening. After Kiatsu, I belched a lot. I belched about 200 times each morning and evening. When there was gas in the stomach, it gave me pain. But after doing Kiatsu and a lot of belches, the pain was gone. Gradually the belching lessened. After one month I was X-rayed again. The ulcers were almost gone and difficult to find the trace. The doctor was astonished and said, "Even a small ulcer is very difficult to get rid of. Normally it is difficult even after six months. A big ulcer like this goes away in one month is incredible." After that when I came back to Japan I had my stomach examined very thoroughly in a big hospital.

They did not even find the traces of any ulcers. It was a very good experience for me to know how powerfully the life power works when it is activated.

22.   Old Pain in the Shoulders

In 1969 I was in Tokyo and had a chance to drink with Mr. Ushiyama, president of YASHICA. While talking with him I found he sometimes put his hand on his right shoulder and rubbed it. I asked him what was the matter and he told me that he used to play baseball when he was young and hurt his shoulder. More than twenty years later he still had pain when it rained. I had him put his arm higher but he could not raise it high enough. He had a little difficulty when he played golf then. I did Kiatsu on his arm for about 20 minutes and he could raise his arm completely without pain. Mr. Ushiyama was very surprised. I explained to him about Ki and two years later when I organized the Ki Society, he donated a lot of money for the foundation.

23.   Contusion

In 1970 an employee of YASHICA was brought to me. During his business trip to southeast Asia, he was attacked by five men. He did not mind being robbed of money, but in the camera there was a very important film. He kept the camera though he was hit and kicked by five men. Fortunately other people came and the attackers ran away. But he could not walk because of the pain. He was sent back to Japan and Mr. Ushiyama, the president of YASHICA sent him to me. By that time he could slowly walk but could not move his upper body even an inch. He could not even move his neck or muscles of his face. I let him sit on a chair and did Kiatsu on his neck and back. First he could move his neck and then he could bend his upper body. After 40 minutes he could move normally. I told him to have an examination at the hospital to make sure. Later he came back and said that the doctor found nothing broken.

24. A Sprained Loin

I had formulated the Ki principles, knew of the existence of Ki, and how to use the power of Ki. By now I felt it pointless to use it only for aikido techniques. In this world it is not of much use merely to teach how to throw people. It is much better to teach people how to control the mind and body. Normally it is healthy people who practice aikido. But there are many people suffering from diseases in the world. It is those people who need to learn mind and body unification. So I organized the Ki No Kenkyukai where I taught only Ki principles. The Ki No Kenkyukai started in September 1971. At that time one of my friends Mr. Toyohara telephoned me. He is a president of a big pharmaceutical shop for medicine in Tokyo and runs a big Japanese restaurant and Shiatsu center with Sauna in Dawny city near Los Angeles. There are 18 Shiatsu therapists working there. When he came back from the U.S.A. he sprained his loin trying to lift his bag at the airport. He had to lie in bed and could not even walk. I had previously cured him of a shoulder pain and he was looking for me to cure his loin. He had to be present for a reception at a newly opened club in Tokyo. I visited him and asked him, "How many hours do you have before you have to be at the reception?" "The reception starts at one o'clock. We have two hours." I said OK and started Kiatsu. After 40 minutes or so I told him to go to the toilet. "No, I cannot even get up from the bed." "Yes, you can." He hesitated but found that he could walk normally. When he came to the reception, all his employees were astonished because they knew he was supposed to be in bed for a few days. Later when I opened a Kiatsu school, Mr. Toyohara asked me to send graduates from there to his Shiatsu center in Dawny.

25. Menstrual Irregularity

I started a Kiatsu therapy group on Wednesday afternoons for people who wanted to receive Kiatsu. Dr. Ariizumi, a director of Ki No Kenkyukai, came as an adviser. Some people had been to several places and found no relief from their problems, so they came to Kiatsu. There were many exceptional cases. One day a woman of 23 came. Her menstruation had stopped for over half a year and the injections from the doctor did not help. Her friends had suggested that she come here. I first asked Dr. Ariizumi who was a gynaecologist to see her. He said that the injections were the only solution. Then I did Kiatsu on her stomach. The stomach was very hard. Normally the femal stomach is soft. I first decided to soften it. Graudally the hard stomach started to separate like the ice on the pond gradually separate in spring. A few days later I did Kiatsu again and the whole stomach became soft. That evening she started to menstruate. Dr. Ariizumi did not understand how it had happened. I also did not understand but my feeling was that the stomach should be soft. I thought the problem was solved. However aftwer twenty days she came again, "Now the menstruation will not stop. It has continued for twenty days." I did Kiatsu again in the same way. The menstruation stopped that day and after that it became normal. The life power works much better than the human wisdom.

26. Migraine Headache (3)

In 1972 I conducted the first Ki seminar in Honolulu. Until then I had only taught aikido in various dojos but this was the first seminar for the general public on the Ki principles. It started with 250 participants. Over the ten days it got more and more successful and by the end there were more than a thousand participants. Dr. John Haward, president of the Luis and

Clark College, Portland, Oregon, was one of these at the seminar. After the seminar when we were talking with several people, he said that there was no way to cure a migraine headache. I said I could cure it. Dr. Haward got interested. He asked me to demonstrate it. In the U.S.A. there are many people suffering from migraines. There are people who suffer from it for ten years or fifteen years. It is possible to ease the pain with medicine but not cure it. The next day Dr. Haward brought with him a woman of 32 or so. She had been born in Hawaii and gone to Los Angeles to get married but had been suffering so badly from migraine headache that she was back home to take a rest. She had a permanent grimace and never seemed to smile. I could not tell whether she was young or old. At first she complained of pain even when I touched her neck. So I transmitted Ki using the barest minimum of pressure so that she did not feel pain. In a little while she did not feel pain even though I started to press more strongly. Eventually the pain was gone even when she moved her neck in every direction. She was very happy and said it was miraculous. When she was happy, she looked very pretty. The pain had been spoiling her beauty. Dr. Haward was astonished. The next year I was invited by the Luis and Clark University to conduct a ten days' seminar. I gave lecture on how to unify the mind and body in the university hall in front of 3,500 audience.

27. Leg

In 1973 on my way to Luis and Clark University for the seminar, I conducted a five days' seminar at the Washington University in Seattle. In most seminars there were always questions about Kiatsu. In Japan few people have heard of Kiatsu but in the U.S.A. many people know the name. Many medical practitioners wanted to know about Kiatsu. At Washington University I taught Kiatsu for one day. Of course in one day I could not explaine everything. I taught only how to extend Ki and how to cure whiplash or migraine headache. After explaining I asked if there were any people there who had physical problems. There were people with headaches, arm, knee, loin problems, etc. I did Kiatsu for ten people in front of hundreds of people. Whereas previously I had taken 30 or 40 minutes to effect a cure, by this time I was much quicker. I took only 5 minutes for each person. All the audience was astonished. Then a beautiful girl of 18 or 19 years old came out hesitatingly and asked me if I could cure her knee. She was always in the front row during the seminar with her leg thrown forward. I always thought she had been born handicapped. She told me she hurt her knee during the practice of karate a year before. When she tried to kick an opponent, the opponent had also kicked. Their legs had collided and the joint of her knee was damaged. She had had an operation but could not bend her knee. The doctor did not know why since he did not sever any tendon or muscle. Later she tried many things to bend her knee, in vain. She gave up physical activity and tried to train her mind. That was why she was taking the seminar. But when she saw the other people being cured, she wondered if her knee also could be cured. After 15 minutes of Kiatsu, she could bend her knee half way. I let her take a rest for a while and then resumed Kiatsu. Then she could walk normally. She was crying for joy. There was great excitement among the audience. She asked me what she should do. I replied, "Your leg is all right now. A pretty girl like you had better not kick others!"

28. Fright

In 1973 after the seminar in New York I flew to Los Angeles to conduct a seminar at California University at Fullerton. The plane was due to stop over at Las Vegas. I had not gone to bed till very late in the previous night because of the farewell party in New York, so I was sleeping on the plane. But

I was waken up by the noise of worried people. The plane was ready to land at Las Vegas but the wheels would not come down and it seemed as if the plane would have to land on its belly. If it caught fire, we might be burned alive. The plane flew a little and started to circle in order to use up all the fuel. I got that information and again fell asleep. If the plane crashed it would not make any difference whether I was asleep or not. If the plane must land on its belly, it would be announced before. I would wake up when it was announced. After a while I woke up with a faint start. An elderly lady sitting beside me told me to look outside giving me an angry look. I looked outside and saw all sorts of fire service cars, police cars, and ambulances. I asked the lady what had happened. She told me they were awaiting in case the plane caught fire. She also told me that the plane had been circling for an hour and half and fortunately they scceeded in getting the wheels to drop. So the plane had landed safely. We had to change plane so everybody tried to get out of the plane as soon as possible. There was no danger at that moment but the workings of the mind prompted people to get out as quickly as possible. As I went out of the plane, I found an elderly lady sitting near the exit very rigid with her eyes rolled up and the whites showing. The only stewardessese were excitedly shouting for the police and an ambulance. I thought that her heart must be beating very quickly. In a consideration of her age, something had to be done immediately. I showed the badge of the San Diego police and asked the stewardess if I could help the lady. I have many badges, as honorary captain of the Honolulu police, New York police, and San Diego Deputy Sheriff. Those badges serve in cases like that. With their consent, I pressed the neck of the lady and first calmed my own breathing and started to control her breathing. In five minutes the rigid body relaxed and the heart beat became calm. The lady opened her eyes and looked around. Then the ambulance came with a stretcher. The lady said she could walk but I whispered to her, "You will not have many chances to ride on a stretcher. Now is a good chance to try it." She nodded and was carried away on it, waving her hand to me. A stewardess thanked me and asked me if I was a doctor. I smiled and said, "Do you know any doctor who does not use medicine?" The stewardess was puzzled.

29. Brain Tumor

For years I have visited the United States to give seminars on Ki. Also I have sent many of my students there and enjoy seeing them on my return visits. Yet for years I avoided going to Europe because I did not wish to interfere with their instructors politics. Then in 1978 we established a Ki No Kenkyukai in Brussels, Belgium and Wales, Great Britain. Soon afterwards I made a trip to Belgium, Germany, France, and Britain to give seminars. It was during my travel in France that I met Mr. Cauhaupe, one of the leading men in their organization. When I met him he had just recovered from a brain tumor operation. Mr. Cauhaupe complained about not feeling well and about losing his balance when he made turns suddenly. Apologetically he refrained from practicing aikido. I then did Kiatsu on his neck and shoulders so that he could move his head freely. Then I taught him how to keep his one point and how to turn without losing his balance. From that point on he continued to practice Ki enthusiastically and earnestly promised to spread the principles of Ki.

30. Cold Feet

From France I flew to Wales to give a seminar at Swansea College. To my surprise there were many students with bad knees. I found that Kiatsu helped temporarily but soon afterwards their legs would swell and the knees would get worse again. Also these students' feet were very cold which is very odd for a whole groupe of young people. In other countries I had never seen these symptoms. Then I examined their college cafeteria diet. All the meals contained foods high in salt content such as ham or bacon. As for potatoes and vegetables, the students often added salt by habit without even tasting the food first. I requested that the students eat less salt and that they do Kiatsu every day. Consequently within one week their knees recovered to normal and their feet became warm.

Chapter 4 Kiatsu Techniques

In the human body there are many nerves passing from the brain through the spinal cord to all parts of the body and the blood circulation passes all through the body. If you put all the small veins together in one line, it would be 96 thousand kilometers which can go round the earth two and a half times. The human body is like a small universe.

The nerve system converges in some places and diverges at other places and harmonizes all functions of the body. It is a very precise machine. What runs this machine? It is called the life power. The universe is one life and human being is a part of it. As long as the life power exists, one is alive and when the life power stops, one dies. So the real health method is to activate this life power. The meeting point of various nerves is called a ganglion. There are many ganglia in the human body. In acupuncture there are difficult names on those points and one must go to school for a few years to learn them. Memorizing those points does not help because the positions of those points move with the posture of the body. It is very difficult to find them exactly.

In Kiatsu Ryoho I only teach the lines. If you run on the high-ways you will surely pass the interchanges. If there is something wrong outside the highway, you can detect it through following the minor roads. Even if the interchanges are all right, if the road itself is damaged, a car cannot run. You must repair both the interchange and the roads.

There are people who treat the foot or the ear when the stomach is wrong. It is true that stomach and feet and ear correspond each other. The human body is one whole unified entity. However when the traffic in one city is blocked, it is useless to repair the road in another city. It is first necessary to send Ki to the damaged part and activate the life power. If the stomach is wrong, first one must fix the stomach and the nerves which controls it, improve the blood circulation for the stomach and activate the life power. This is the treatment of Kiatsu Ryoho.

The best way is to do Kiatsu on the whole body and to activate the life power of the whole body. But one cannot take time to treat the whole body. One must practice to do Kiatsu as little as possible in a short time and cure the disease exactly. If one masters the correct techniques and the correct way of extending Ki, one will not get tired even doing Kiatsu for ten or twenty people everyday. Even if one gets tired, one can recover easily by Ki breathing.

1. Backbone

The brain gives messages to the body and these messages pass through the backbone. If the backbone is good, the intestines are well-protected. If some part of the internal organs is wrong, the backbone will show it. So I will first explain the spinal cord.

In the middle of the back is the backbone. Press on the line beside the backbone and change the direction of the fingertip toward the inside of the bone. Do not press on the bone. It is very dangerous to press the back-bone itself because it would move the vertebra and damage the nerve on the backbone. This line is called line A. The patient will be able to feel this line when Kiatsu is done to it and feel very well. If the body is fatigued, press on the lines A and A'. The fatigue will go away immediately.
The left part of the body is A, B, C, etc. and the right parts is A', B', C' etc. Next there is a big line along the backbone about one inch away from it.

This is called line B. This line approaches the backbone at the neck and continues down a little further away from it and again approaches the backbone at the hip and goes down along the line A. When some part of the internal organs is wrong, it shows on this B line. When something is the matter with the stomach, press the B line which corresponds to the stomach. The patient will be able to feel it by himself.

(photo 9)

Beside the line B, line C runs from the back to the belly toward the one point in the lower abdomen.

(photo 10)

Line D passes the back part of the shoulder blade, runs along it and reaches the side. Line E runs sideways on the shoulder blade.

(photo 8)

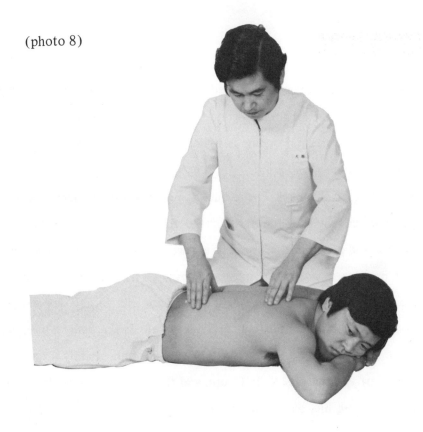

(photo 9)

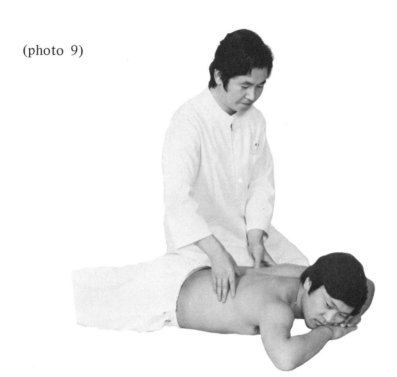

(photo 10)

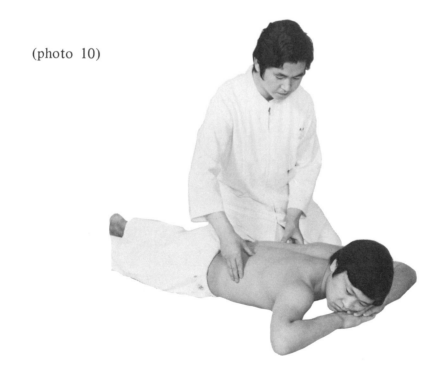

(photo 11)

A   baseball pitcher often hurts this E line or D line. When the patient is weak, first make the neck and shoulders soft and then press well on lines A and B.

(Fig. 4)

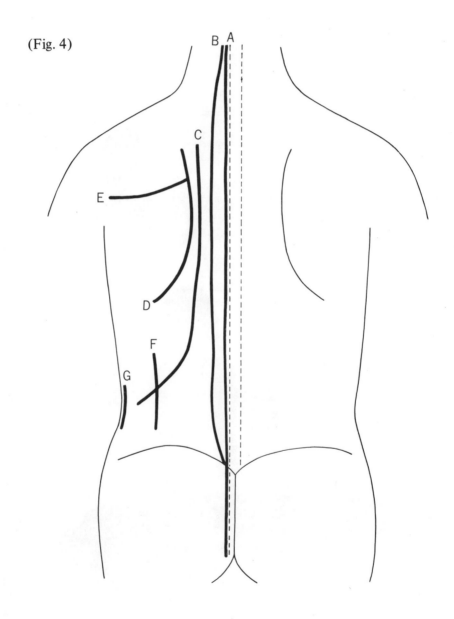

(photo 11)

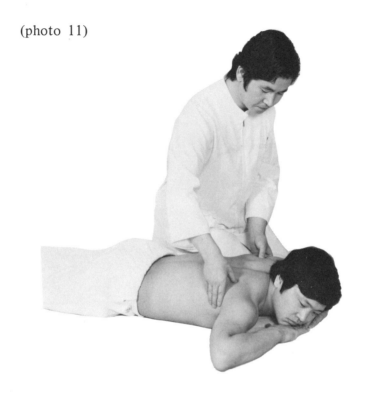

2. Hip

There are many people suffering from sciatica. The patient must sit down with his legs thrown forward. First press the B line from the shoulders to the hip. Then press the upper edge of the hipbone downward. This is line A of the hip.

(photo 12)

Then press line B of the hip upward to the hipbone.

(figure 6)

Then check the lines C and D and find the damaged part. If you find the damaged line, press there intently. Then sit behind the patient and press

(Fig. 5)

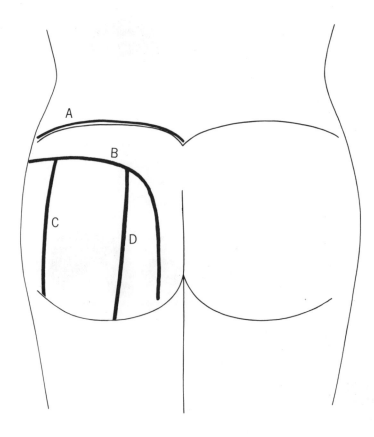

the B and B' lines of the back with thumbs to send Ki while the patient bends his body forward as much as possible. (photo 13)

Next keep the thumbs on the same points and let the patient bend his body backward as much as possible. (photo 14)

(photo 12)

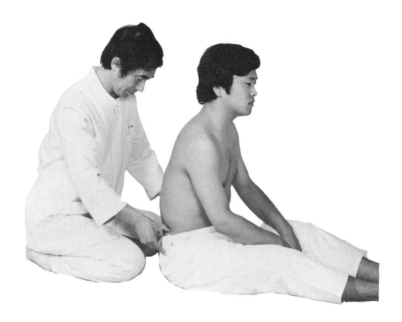

(Fig. 6)

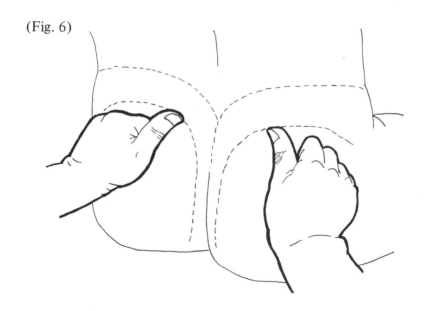

(photo 13)

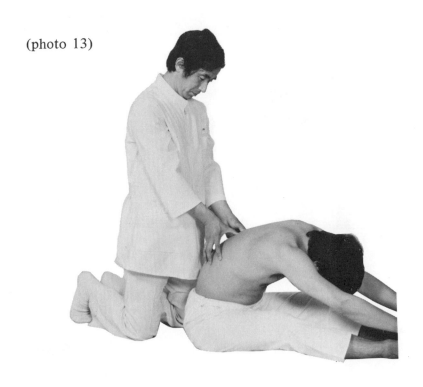

(photo 14)

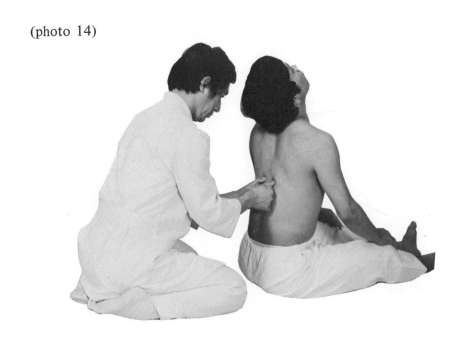

Then change the position of the thumbs a little down and do the same. The patient will not be able to bend much in the beginning but as you continue Kiatsu, he will improve a great deal. Next hold the patient's shoulder with the right hand and have him twist his body toward the right as much as possible and press the line B of the back with your left thumb. (photo 15) Do the same with the other side. Then press line B, C, and D of the hip while the patient moves forward and backward and right and left. If you find a place where the patient feels a particular pain, keep him in that position and send Ki to the place longer. Then ask the patient to stand up and try all the movements. If he can move without pain, he is already cured. A person who came supported by someone else will be able to go back walking normally.

(photo 15)

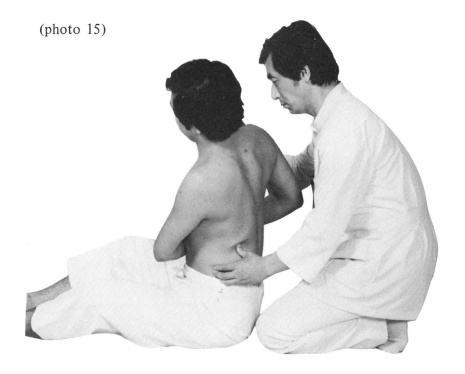

3. Leg

There are eight lines in the leg. When standing erect, line A runs down the middle of the thigh along the bone of the lower leg and reaches the middle toe of the foot. Line B runs along the outside of the leg. Line C runs down the back side of the leg.

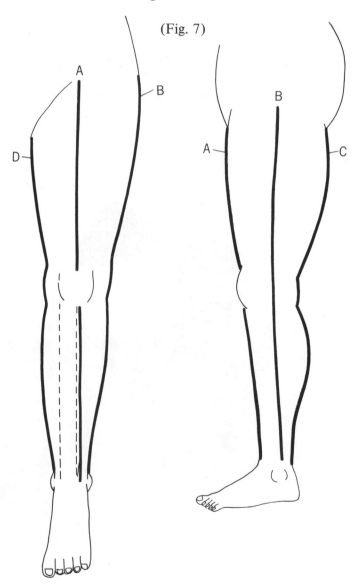

(Fig. 7)

(figures 7 and 8)

Line E runs between lines A and B, line F runs between lines B and C, and line G runs between lines C and D, and line H runs between lines D and A.

(Fig. 8)

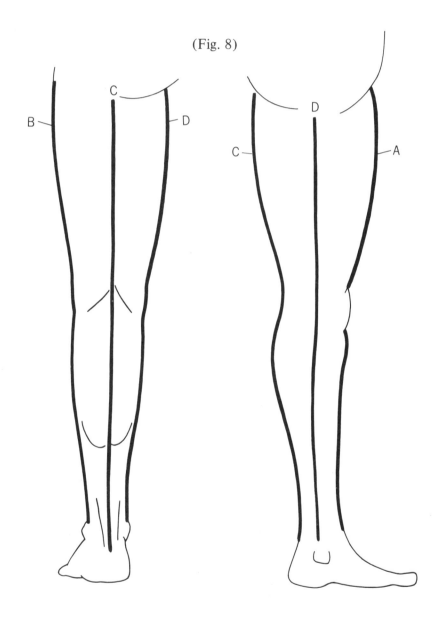

(figures 9 and 10)

These eight lines are main lines. There are smaller lines coming out of them.
It is not necessary to press all eight lines. Just press the necessary lines which

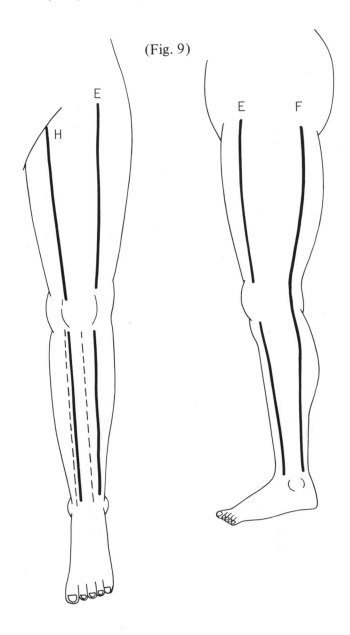

(Fig. 9)

correspond the disease or the problem. However, when the blood circulation is not good and the feet are cold, you have to press all the major lines to activate the life power of the whole leg. The difficulty is to find the line in the thigh because of the big muscles there. The same problem lies with lines C and D of the hip.

(Fig.10)

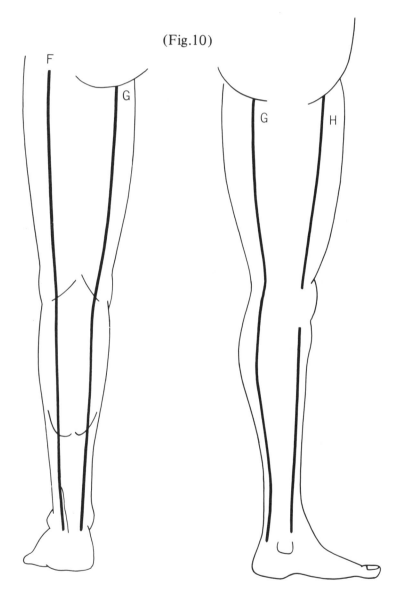

(photo 16)

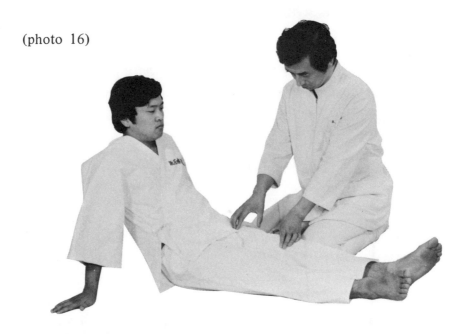

The patient sits with his legs thrown forward. First press the muscles of the leg so that the muscle does not move. With the other hand find the line. (photo 16)

If the problem is on the back side of the leg, let the patient lie on his stomach and find the line in the same way. Otherwise it is very difficult to find the line because the muscle moves so that you cannot press perpendicularly toward the center. The patient will also be frustrated because the Ki does not come in. If you press the line correctly, the patient will feel the Ki coming in and be content. Once you find the line, do not let it escape. When you move your finger, first keep the line with one hand and move the other hand to catch the line and then move the former hand. In this way you can press all the lines without losing them. The lines F, C, and G in the calf are also difficult to find. Try to find them in the same manner.

Line C and D of the hip are also difficult to find. If you just knead, you will not be able to touch the line. If you just press, you will not catch the line because the muscles moves and changes the direction of your finger.

There are people who say they have no pain when being pressed with fingers but have a strong pain while walking. It is impossible that they do not have pain when pressed. It is only because you did not yet find the line. You must hold the place with one hand and find the C and D lines with the other hand. Then you can surely find the point which gives pain. Do Kiatsu there and the patient will be cured.

4. Neck

Line A of the neck is hidden behind the cervical vertebrae and continues to line A of the back. Further away from the vertebrae runs line B of the neck which continues to the line B of the back. Line C runs to the shoulder blade. Line D runs from behind the ear and line E runs down from the front of the ear. Line F runs from the chin to the throat and line G runs down the side of the Adam's apple.

(figures 11, 12, and 13)

(Fig. 11)

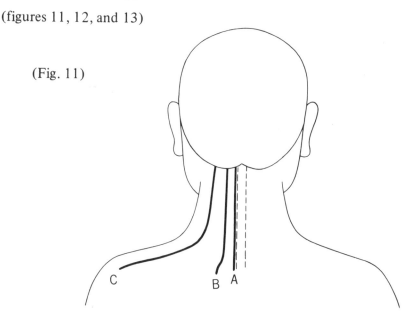

(Fig. 12)

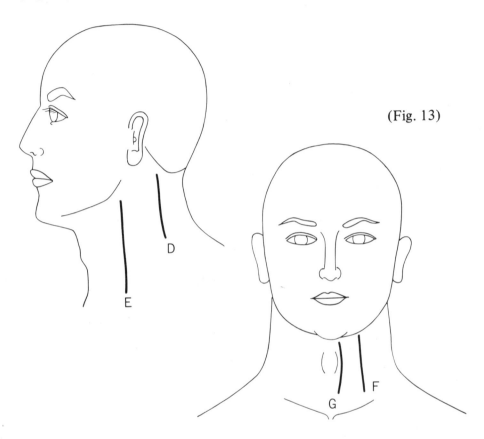

(Fig. 13)

It is said that migraine headaches cannot be cured. Medicine can only stop the pain temporarily. Whiplash also takes a long time to cure. Both pertain to the lines A, B, and C of the neck. When these lines get soft and flexible, they can be cured easily. A human being always uses his brain. Naturally the blood tends to stay in the head and the shoulders stiffen. So once one gets migraine headache or whiplash, the problems are compounded, so it is very difficult to recover by oneself. That is why someone else must send Ki to him and activate his life power. Once it recovers, the life power can manage alone in curing the problem.

(1) How to cure a migraine headache

First ask the patient to bend his head in all directions. Normally the patient will not be able to bend well. Do Kiatsu on lines A, B, and C of the neck. Place yourself higher than the patient when pressing the neck and shoulders. If the patient sits on the floor, sit on a chair. If the patients sits on a chair, stand behind the chair. If both are the same height, your arms are higher than the shoulders so you tend to use physical strength and easily get tired. It is preferable that your hand is lower than your shoulder and sends Ki downward to the patient.

(photo 17)

(photo 17)

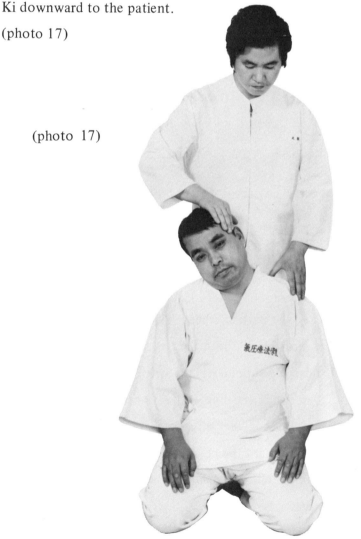

75

(photo 18)

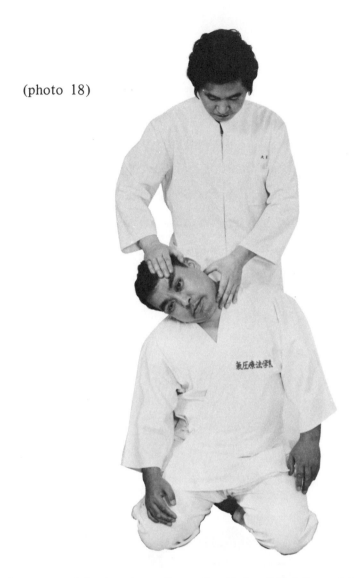

Put your right hand on the patient's head lightly and let the head bend to the right as much as possible without forcing it. Press the soft part on the end of the line C near the shoulder blade with your left thumb. After pressing there 10 or 20 seconds the line will get softer and the head can bend more. The patient will not feel any pain. Change the position of the thumb along the line C toward the head. By the time the thumb reaches the head, the patient will be able to bend his head till the head touches the right shoulder. (photo 18)

(photo 19)

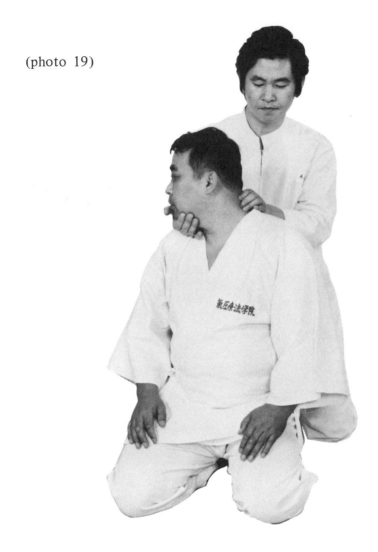

Repeat this on the right side so that the patient can bend to the left completely.

Next press line B with your three middle fingers. Put your right hand on the patient's chin and turn his face to the right. Then find the hard line on the left side of the neck and press it with your left fingers. At first the patient will not be able to turn his neck well but with Kiatsu he will be able to turn until the chin comes to the line of the right shoulder. (photo 19)

(photo 20)

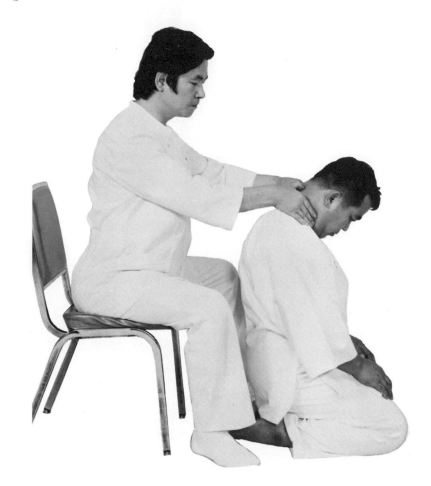

Do the same on the other side. Bend the patient's head forward and press line B with both thumbs from the head to the shoulders. (photo 20)

Press once down the length of line B, then next time let the patient bend his head forward and backward while being pressed. (photo 21)

(photo 21)

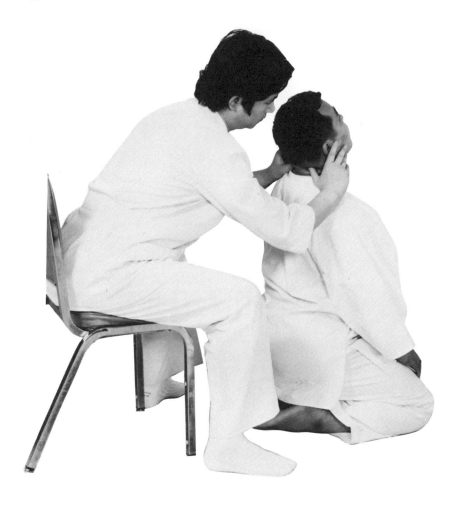

By this time the patient can move freely in all directions. Then ask the patient to move his neck freely as you press line B, B' C, and C'. If the patient feels pain in some particular position, keep his neck in that position and press there.

(photo 22)

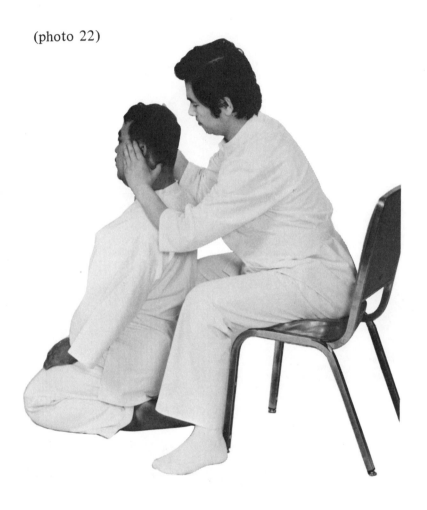

Hold the patient's forehead with your right hand and press along the line F upward toward the inside of the brain with left thumb. (figure 14) The patient will feel pain penetrating toward the forehead. (photo 22) When the brain aches, the skull hinders the Ki penetration. So it is easier to send Ki into the brain on the line F. The patient will feel very light in the head.

Next hold the patient's head with the right hand and press place E with the left three fingers. (figure 15)

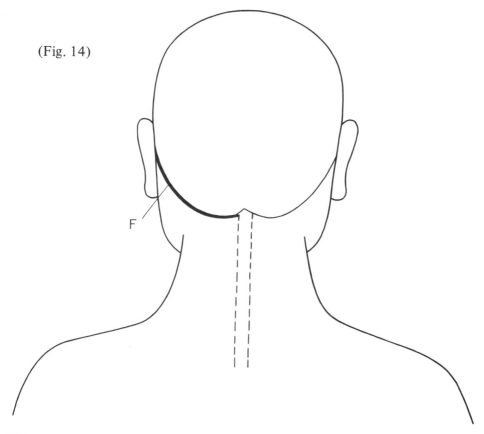

(Fig. 14)

F

This point E is an area, not a line. This is a nerve center. First the patient will not feel much pain. But as you continue Kiatsu, he will gradually feel more pain. Press all over the E point. When the forehead aches or the eyes are not clear, press there. In this way the migraine headache can be cured. If it is not be cured at once, repeat once each day for 3 or 4 days and most headaches will be cured.

When one catches a cold, sometimes one feels cold or pain even when someone else touches one's hair. It will go away when the cold is over but occasionally one has a pain outside the skull with no reason. In that case press lines A, B, C, and D of the head and find the painful point. Then press there. (figure 16 and 17)

(Fig. 15)

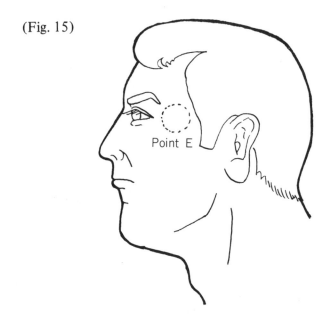

Point E

(2) Whiplash

In the case of whiplash point E of the head is not necessary. The rest is the same as the migraine headache. In the case of whiplash it is better to press line B of the back down to the middle of the back. And do not forget to press while bending the patient's neck forward and backward. If necessary, also press line A of the neck, but normally it is not necessary.

(3) Stiff Shoulders

As one gets old it is common to have problems in the loins or shoulders. It is due to incorrect posture which results in fatigue. Press lines A, B, and C of the neck and lines B, C, D, and E of the back. When you find the stiff part, press there well. Sometimes not only the lines but also the muscles are stiff and weak. In that case press the muscle lightly for a long time. The muscle fatigue gives dull pain even if one does not use it. This dull pain may

(Fig. 16)

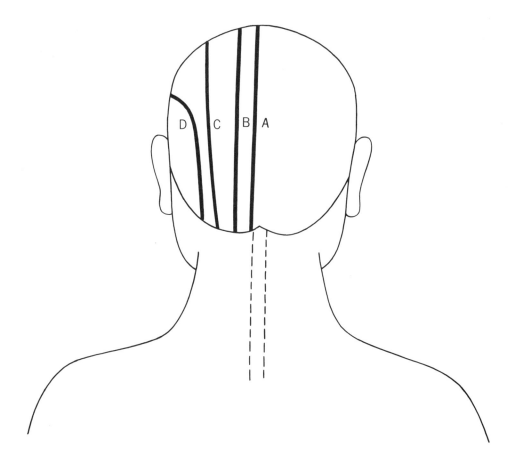

(Fig. 17)

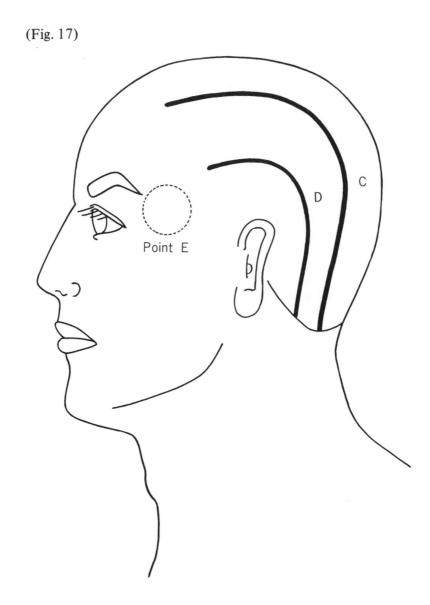

Point E

D

C

disturb sleep. Use Kiatsu on the muscle for a long time and take away the fatigue.

5. Chest

Line A runs along the upper side of the clavicle. Then there are lines between the ribs from line B to line J. (figure 18) After being hit in the chest or influenza, one sometimes have a pain in his chest. This is normally called pleurodynia. When one tries to breathe in deeply, his chest hurts and he cannot inhale. Many people think it is due to the heart. If the heart stops, one is dead. So of course it is disturbing. First press all the lines of the chest by yourself. You will find a particularly painful place. Press there calmly. At first one will have a lot of pain but as the Kiatsu continues, the pain will subside. Then keep your finger on the point and inhale as deeply as possible. The chest will not hurt even with the deep breath. Breathe out smoothly and breath in smoothly. Repeat this four or five times and then breathe without the finger. If you can breathe deeply without pain and swing the arms freely without pain, your chest is all right. After all this, if the pain still continues, go to the hospital and get examined. Normally Kiatsu will be sufficient. With a heart problem, do Kiatsu on the shoulders and back, and do Ki breathing well. It will naturally be cured.

(Fig. 18)

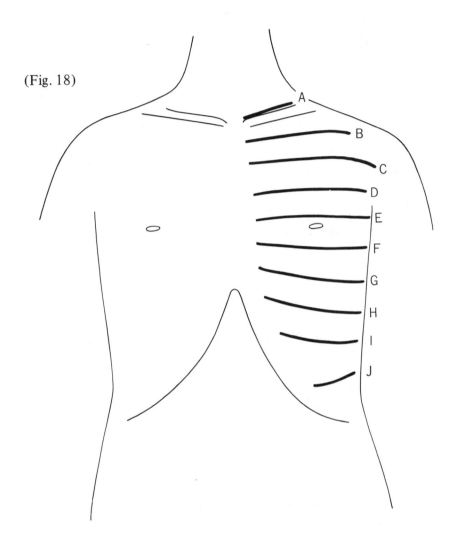

6. Stomach

From the pit of the stomach to the end of the lower abdomen runs line A. A and A' lines are the same in this case.

Lines B, C, D run parallel at the distance of about four centimeters. Try with your own stomach and you will easily find those lines because you feel good when those lines are pressed. (figures 19)

(Fig. 19)

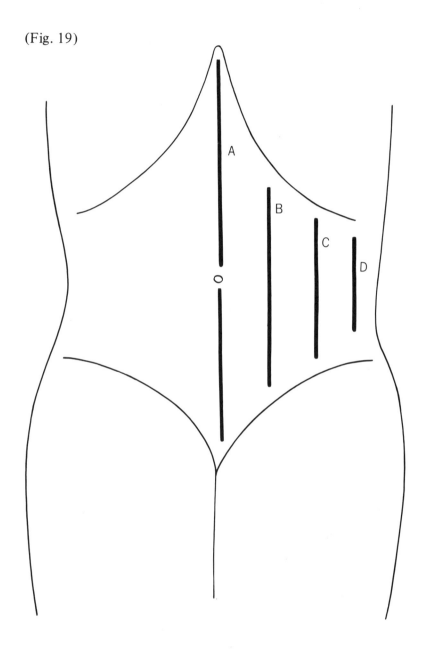

When the stomach or intestines indicate a problem, press all the lines A, B, C, and D lines. The internal organs are all connected so the problem of one part influences the other parts. The first round one should press line A downward, then Line B' upward, and line B downward. This is the direction of the food passing through the intestines. Once you press this cycle, you can press anywhere you like. Press the hard or painful places. But do not press the navel. For unknown reasons pressing there does not feel good. It is better not press places that don't feel good. Sometimes you will find people who have no pulse in the stomach or intestines. Their intestines are not functioning well. They always feel heavy in their stomach and intestines. In that case press one place for a long time until you can feel a pulse. Count the pulse while doing Kiatsu. When one presses at one place for a long time, sometimes his Ki stops. But as long as one is counting the pulse, one's Ki continues. Then the pulse will become strong. In the case of a stomach ulcer or constipation, continue Kiatsu at one place for more than one hundred pulses. You can use the thumbs or the three middle fingers together. There are people whose pulse is abnormally strong in the intestines. In that case while doing Kiatsu the pulse will become calmer. Do not knead the stomach. It is very dangerous since it could twist the intestines. Kiatsu is not dangerous because you do not move the fingers but only extend Ki. First press very calmly and as the stomach becomes softer the fingers naturally penetrate deeper. In the case of a woman's disease, press the lower abdomen calmly. Even if one has no problem, by doing Kiatsu before going to bed and after waking up in the morning, one promotes health and never becomes constipated. When one eats something bad, the whole digestive system will ache. In that case do Kiatsu all over, and the pain will subside. Go to the toilet as often as possible. After getting rid of everything which should go out of the bowels, one can easily recover. One must repeat Kiatsu until everyting goes out. When one has appendicitis, first try Kiatsu. If the pain subsides one does not need an operation and will surely recover. If the pain still continues, then go to hospital. Doing 20 or 30 minutes Kiatsu will not make it too late. There are many people who have received unnecessary operations. Some doctors say the appendix is unnecessary. It is only human beings who have not yet discovered its function. Sumo people often say if one cuts out the appendix, he loses power. It is better not to have an operation for its removal.

7. Arm

When the arm is naturally hanging down, line A runs from the center of the shoulder to the middle finger. Line B runs to the small finger and line C runs down the other side of line A. Line D runs from the front of the shoulder to the thumb. (figure 20) Between lines A, B, C, and D run lines E, F, G, and H. There are 8 main lines, just like the leg. (figure 21)

(1) Shoulder

Some people cannot lift their arm or move it behind because of the pain in the shoulders. After a dislocation, the joint can be fixed easily, but sometimes the arm doesn't move freely. It is because the tendons and muscles which were damaged have not healed. The bone can mend after one or two weeks if it is broken and the dislocated joint can be fixed in a few days. But the damaged tendons take more time. By doing Kiatsu on the tendons and muscles, one will be able to use the arm immediately. When the bone is broken, it is better not to touch it for one or two weeks until the broken part is set into place. If you touch it and the broken part slips out of its proper place, it will heal incorrectly. In the case of shoulders, the important lines are lines A, E and H. First press these three lines down to the elbow.

(Fig. 20)

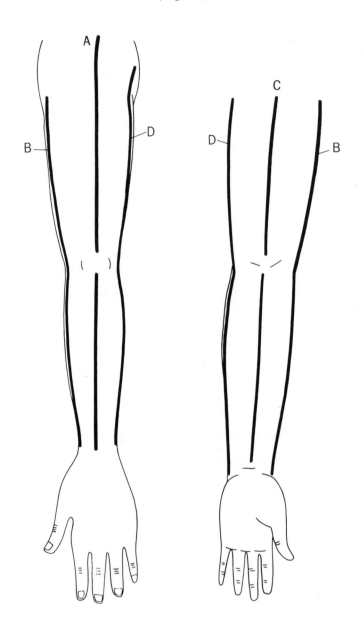

(Fig. 21)

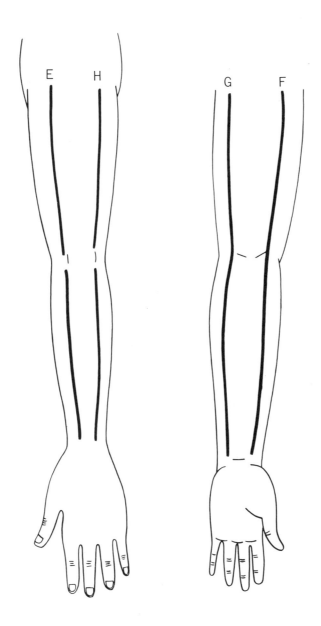

(photo 23)

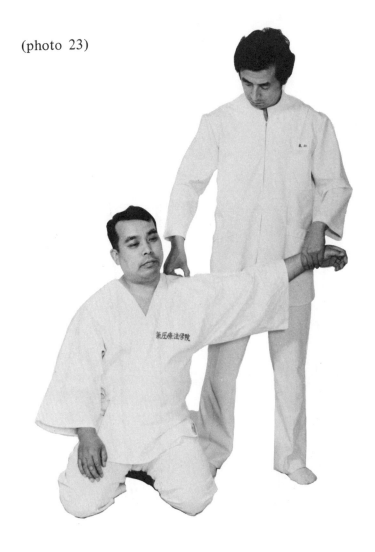

Then press the left shoulder on line A with the right thumb while lifting the patient's left hand as high as possible (photo 23). As the shoulder becomes softer, the arm can be gradually raised. Change the position of the right thumb till it reaches the upper arm. Then go back to the shoulder . By repeating this, the arm will go all the way up. Keep the arm stretched upward and do Kiatsu (photo 24).

(photo 24)

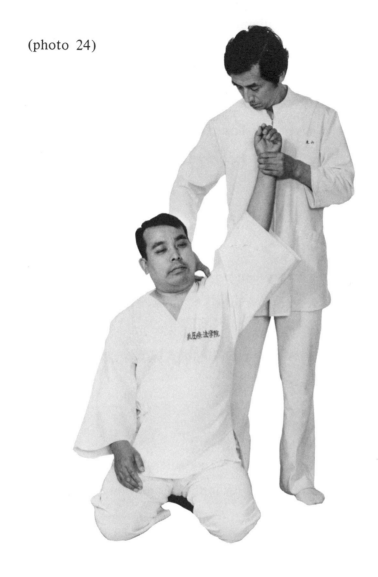

When you put the patient's left arm down, keep the right thumb on line A and put the arm down calmly. After the arm is completely down, take off the thumb. If you take off the thumb first and let the arm down, the tendon can be damaged, because the stiff tendon is stretched and not yet in harmony with the other tendons and muscles. It is very important to put the arm down keeping the tendon fixed with the right thumb. After putting the patient's arm down calmly, let him move the arm by himself. The arm can go up as far as it had gone with the help of the therapist. When the arm is painful in movement to the front, let him stretch his arm forward and press lines B and H in the back of the shoulder. When the arm cannot go behind, gently hold it behind and press line H. Lastly, ask the patient move his arm freely and if he finds some position painful, press while his arm is in that position.

(2) Upper arm

In the case of neuralgia of the upper arm, normally press lines A, B, D, E, and H. Some elderly people have weak life power in the muscle itself and complain of dull pain in the muscle. In that case press all the muscles. The neuralgia of elderly people is sometimes due to the weak life power of the muscle.

(3) Elbow

When the elbow is damaged, ask the patient where the pain is. Also ask how he damaged it, and put his elbow in that position to find the line. When shihonage, an aikido art, is executed by an unskilled person, the elbow can be damaged. Press the elbow at lines B or F and bend the elbow in the position of shihonage. You will find the painful point. You must find the correct place since doing Kiatsu on the wrong place is not useful. Do Kiatsu on the correct place while keeping the elbow in the position of shihonage (photo 25). Then stretch and bend the arm. After Kiatsu ask the patient to od the same movement. If he feels no pain, it is cured. This kind of problem can be corrected immediately

(photo 25)

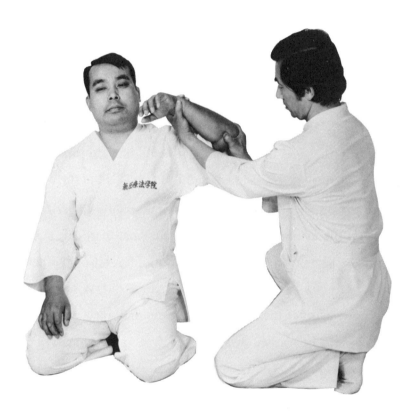

(4) Wrist

When one falls down on his wrists or by receiving an improperly applied aikido art like nikkyo or kotegaeshi, his wrists can be damaged. Ask the patient where the pain is and bend the wrist in the position when it was damaged to find the most painful place. If you do not find the correct place, it is useless to do Kiatsu. Once you find the correct place, one can cure it immediately.

8. Eye

Line A runs horizontally along the eyebrow where the bone protrudes. Line B also runs horizontally under the bone. Place your finger between line B and the eyball to find a line which elicits pain. This is line C. Close the eyes and do Kiatsu all over the eyeball. This is place D.

When one closes his eyes, the eye lashes become line E. Under the eyeball runs line F (figure 22). When one has a headache because of bad eyesight, do Kiatsu not only the lines of the head and neck, but also line A of the eyes. When the eyes are tired, press line B and C. Place D is the surface of the eyeball, so do not press there. Just put the three middle fingers together and place them on the eye-ball softly. If there are small particles in the back of the eyelids, do Kiatsu on place D. In ten minutes, all of the particles will be absorbed. If pus has formed, it will all come out. After that put clean water in a bowl and put the face into the water and open and close the eyes. All of the pus will be washed away. In the case of inflammation of the eyelids, do Kiatsu on line E. The swelling will gradually reduce. If a sticky secretion collects in the eyes, it may take a few days to be cured. Both the inflammation of the eylids and the trachoma can be cured in 3 or 4 days by doing ten minutes interval of Kiatsu 2 or 3 times a day. Even if you have nothing wrong, if you study too much or get too tired in the eyes, do Kiatsu on the lines B and C to take away the fatigue. If you have weak eyesight, continue Kiatsu on lines A, B, and C. Your eyesight will improve tremendously.

(Fig. 22)

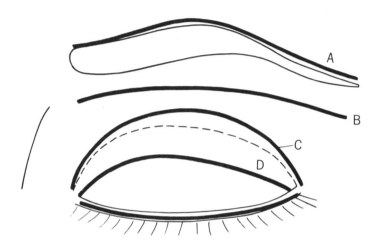

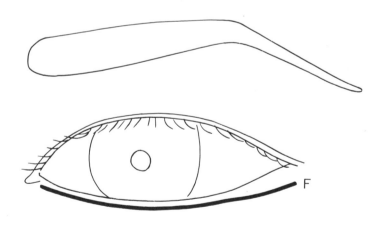

9. Nose

Line A runs downward beside the bridge of the nose. Line B runs down at the bottom of the nose. Line C goes beside the line B toward the ear (figure 23). When the nose is hit hard for some reason, one must send Ki to the damaged place and along line A. The pain will go away sooner and there will not be problems later. Coryza is very difficult to cure in hospital. Do Kiatsu on lines B and C many times. Line C must be pressed upward from the under-side of the cheekbone with the tuhmb. In the case of a stuff nose, do Ki-atsu on line C. When a baby has a stuffy nose, it has difficulty sleeping. When the baby falls asleep, put the fingertip on the line C lightly. The baby will have clear nose and it can fall into a deep sleep. Usually a baby will not let you do Kiatsu while it is awake.

(Fig. 23)

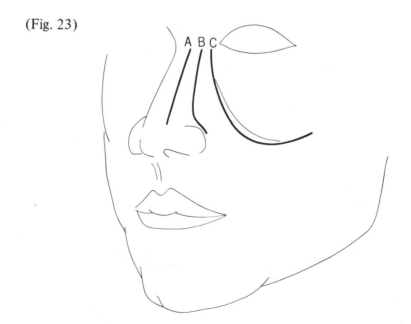

10. Mouth

Line A runs sideways on the upper gum. Line B runs under line A on the point where the teeth come out of the gum. Line C is the line where the teeth come out of the lower gum. Line D runs along the lower gum to the ear (figure 24).

If you have a toothache, go to the dentist. It is very difficult to extend Ki into the teeth. So it is better to see a dentist. However when you have a toothache in the middle of the night, the dentist will not treat you immediately . He will tell you to come the next day and you will have to suffer all night. At that time do Kiatsu on the point which gives you pain. You do not have to put your fingers into your mouth. Just do Kiatsu from the outside. The pain will subside and you will be able to go to sleep. If it starts aching again, do Kiatsu again. Then go to the dentist as soon as possible. You can recover very quickly because you have a lot of life power. When one has pain around his chin so that he cannot chew or laugh, do Kiatsu on line D near the ear.

(Fig. 24)

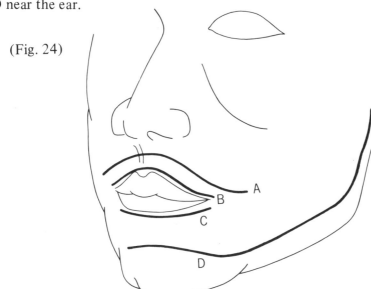

11. Ear

When one has pain in the ear or has a difficulty in hearing, press line A and B often (figure 25). However when there is an acute pain, it is better to go to the hospital to get a close examination since there could be many serious problems. After being treated at the hospital, if the problem persists, try Kiatsu many times to recover the life power. Even if you can stop the pain with Kiatsu, it is better to see a doctor to make sure that it is not serious . Do not press under the ear since it creates an unpleasant sensation.

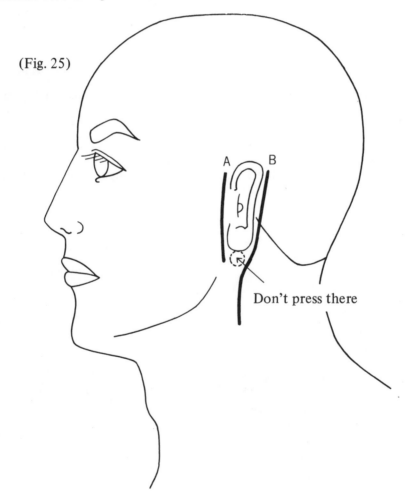

(Fig. 25)

Don't press there

12. Throat

When one catches a cold and has a throat pain, press lines G and G' of the neck with the thumb and the middle finger. After this press lines F and F'. Same treatment is useful in laryngitis. (figure 13)

When one has a cold and a pain in the chest, it is possible to have bronchitis. In that case put the middle finger to the soft place where the two collar bones meet and do Kiatsu downward to send Ki inside the chest. Also do Kiatsu on each line of the chest. For asthma, first take away the stiffness of the neck and the shoulders. Then do Kiatsu on lines G and F and lines A, B, and C of the chest. Then let the patient do Ki breathing. The patient can surely overcome the problem.

13. Finger

When one has a sprained finger, first pull the finger strongly. The sprained finger can result in a deformed joint. When the joint is deformed and heals, the finger can never bend. Pull the finger well and the joint will fall into place with a little cracking sound. Do not forget to pull it to make sure that it heals properly. Line A goes from the middle of the nail to the base of the finger. Line B along the outside of the finger, line C is on the opposite side of line A and line D, opposite side of line B. Lines E, F, G, and H run between the lines A, B, C, and D (figure 26).

Press lines B and D at the joint with your thumb and the middle finger and bend the finger gradually. Later the patient should be able to bend his finger completely. Keep your fingers on the lines B and D and stretch the finger, then take your finger off. Next do Kiatsu on the line A to bend the finger in the other direction.

(Fig. 26)

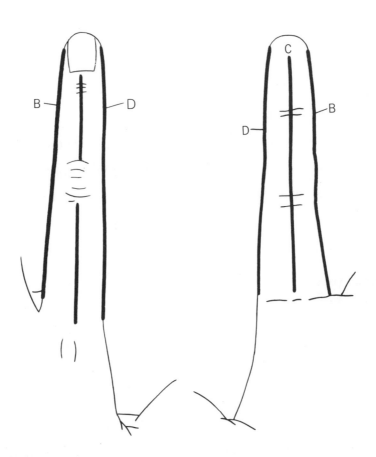

Then press lines E and H. It is not especially necessary to press on lines C, F, and G, but all the other lines should be pressed well. When the patient bends and stretches his fingers without pain, they are cured. In the case of a fester under the nail, do not press the painful part but just touch it lightly and extend Ki. It will take some time until the pain subsides. Fester under the nail can be removed by a doctor but it will often reoccur. If you cure it with Kiatsu, it will never reoccur. Do the same with the toes. When the back of the hand aches, press the side of the bones which correspond to the finger.

14. Knee

(Fig. 27)

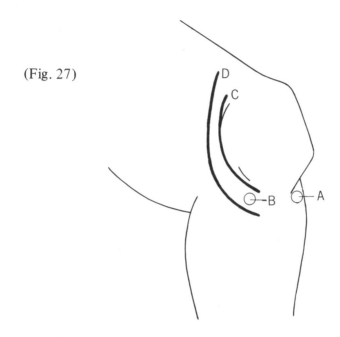

When one hurts his knees, he has difficulty walking or kneeling down. The knees are normally very difficult to cure. Sometimes one does not have pain when the knees are pressed upon or massaged but has an acute pain when walking or bending. That is why many people think something is wrong with the inside of the joint. So they think it should be operated upon. However, most knee problems can be solved without an operation. It is only necessary to find the correct places. There are two soft points, A and B, just under the knees (figure 27). Do Kiatsu on these points A and B with the two thumbs while the patient's knee is half bent. First the patient will not feel pain but as you continue extending Ki, points A and B get softer and the patient will start feeling pain (photo 26).

Keep the thumbs on the two spots and let the patient stretch his legs calmly.

(photo 26)

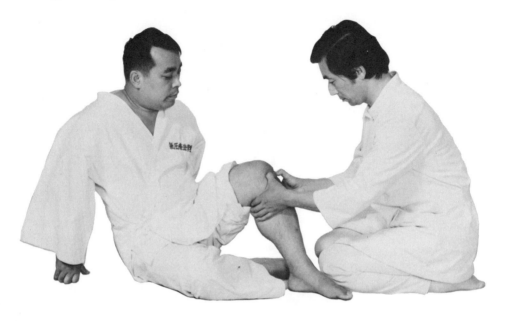

When the leg is almost stretched, the therapist can feel a small line at the points A and B. When the thumbs touch the small line the patient will feel a very strong pain. They are the correct lines. Normally people cannot find them (photo 27). Then keep the thumbs on the spots and ask the patient to bend his knee until his foot touches his buttocks (photo 28). While the patient bends and stretches his knee many times, keep the thumbs on the spots. If necessary do Kiatsu on lines C and D. Sometimes the lines E and H of the leg are stiff, which makes the knee difficult to bend. In that case do Kiatsu on the lines E and H near the knee. If the patient kneels on his knees and the bottocks do not touch the feet, do Kiatsu on spots A and B as the patient tries to lower his buttocks. The patient will be able to kneel down completely. When the patient can sit down and stand up with ease, the knee is cured.

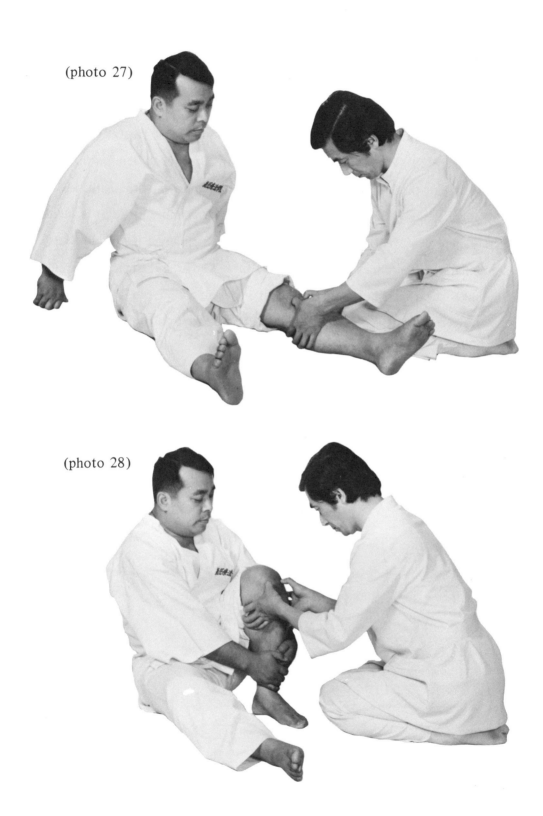

(photo 27)

(photo 28)

15. Ankle

When his ankle is sprained, ask the patient where the pain is. Do Kiatsu on lines A, B, C, and D so that the patient can bend his ankle freely in all directions (figure 28). When the foot cannot be stretched, do Kiatsu on the lines at the side of the bones which correspond to the toes while the ankle is well stretched. If the patient can stand on the toes of his injured foot, it is cured. The patient can even run after an ankle has been sprained if you do Kiatsu immediately. Sometimes there is no pain after Kiatsu, but the next morning the ankle swells and becomes painful. It is due to a damaged line which had not received Kiatsu. You must do Kiatsu on that line. If the bone is broken it is better to see a doctor.

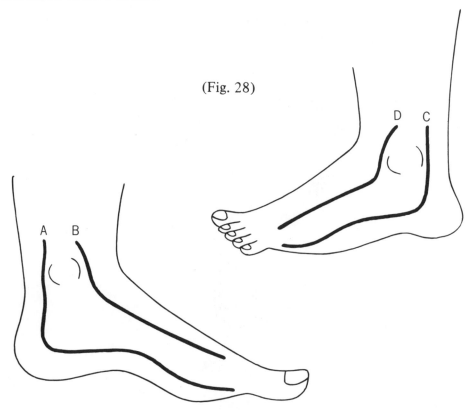

(Fig. 28)

16. Fester

Sometimes parts of the body can fester. After the pus comes out, the pain is relieved. But before that when the festered part is red, it is very painful. In that case you cannot touch the part immediately. Keep your fingers a short distance away from the skin and send Ki. Naturally the finger goes closer to the skin and finally touches it. In this way the patient will not feel pain since the Ki touches first. Keep your finger there and the festering part will become softer and your finger can penetrate into it naturally without giving pain to the patient. When the finger passes the festering part and arrives at the part under the pus, take off the finger calmly and press the next point. Start from the surrounding area and go in circle approaching the center. After one and half circle, the weakest point in the center will break and the pus will come out. A hollow will remain when the pus is pressed out. Leave the core in the center and the next day apply Kiatsu again, this time pressing the core out. During this process the patient will not feel much pain. If the therapist tries to press out the core immediately, there will be pain. That is why it is better to wait until the next day.

17. Breast

After a baby is born, sometimes the mother's milk will not come. Even if she goes to the hospital and gets injection, sometimes it still does not come out. In that case send Ki to the breasts in the same way as the fester. Then naturally the milk will come out.

18. Nosebleed

When the patient's nose start bleeding, stuff his nose and have him lie down on his back for ten minutes or so. The bleeding will naturally stop.

However when he is working, walking, or doing something else he cannot lie down for ten minutes. In that case there is a method to stop the bleeding immediately. Let the patient sit down with a towel on his nose. Hold the patient's forehead with your left hand and put your right hand on line A of the patient's neck in the middle of his neck and concentrate there (photo 29). Swing up your right hand (photo 30) and hit the neck of the patient

(photo 29)

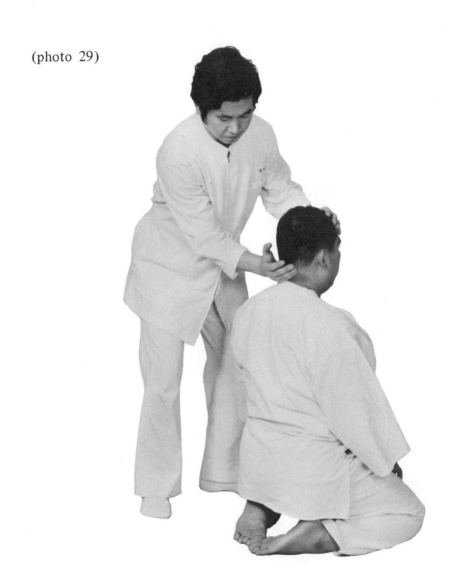

twice in a row with a shout of "i-yea-i". The bleeding will stop immediately. It is important to know how to hit twice successively. If you only hit once, you might give him pain. The strength of the strike must be carefully adjusted. If the hit is too strong, the bleeding might stop but the patient will have a whiplash. By hitting twice with one shout, you will only give the patient shock without pain. Try it first on your own left arm. If you hit only once, you will feel pain. By hitting twice letting your hand bounce, you will

(photo 30)

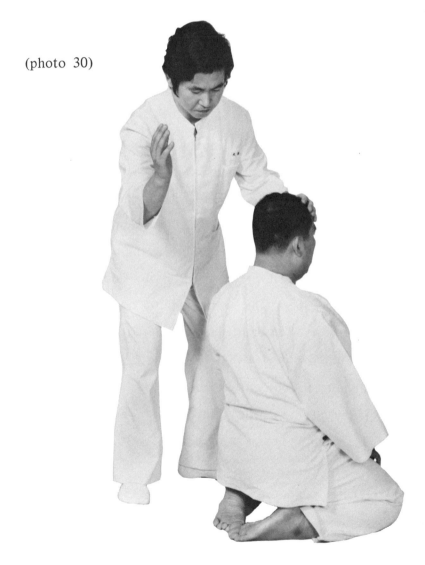

not give pain. If you create a pain when you hit your own arm, do not hit another person's neck.

The rationale for this blow-to-the-neck method may be clarified by drawing analogy to a war time air raid alert. When an air attack is imminent, a siren is sounded to alert the people to take cover. All unnecessary activities are terminated, even production work is shut down because at the time of the emergency alert, it is not regarded as important. Only essential activities are allowed, especially those involved in preparation for the impending attack and resulting damages, e.g., operation of antiaircraft batteries or the manning of first aid stations. When the all-clear siren is sounded, the emergency operations are relaxed and normal activities are again allowed. In the similar manner, a blow to the neck is a shock-signal that there is an attack occurring to the person and there will most probably be an injury sustained to the body. When the brain received the shock-signal, it alerts the whole body to prepare for disaster. It means important organs like the heart and liver must increase their activity, so additonal blood supply is pumped there. Operations unnecessary for the emergency such as the activity of the lining of the nasal passage is closed down for an instant by shutting off the blood supply to the capillaries there. This action stops the nose bleed even though it is not a real emergency. The brain notices the lack of danger and removes the alert signal but in the reflex reaction, the bleeding has stopped.

If the first attempt does not work, the hitting was too weak to alert the patient. Try once again with a little bit harder strike. You must give a shock to the patient. The shout also helps to give a shock.

19. Kappo

If an individual sustains a severe shock in the abdomen, drowns or is electrocuted, he loses consciousness and stops breathing. If he is left in this state of delicate balance between life and death, he may easily die. It is of dire necessity to arouse him. This procedure is called Kappo. In a situation where a person stops breathing, the important thing is restoring the first breath since subsequent breaths follow automatically. There are many methods called Kappo, but the most popular is the method of raising the upper body of the patient and placing your own knee on the backbone. Holding the shoulders with both hands, pull them to open the chest. This method is effective when the situation is not too serious. For example, if one receives a punch in the stomach and stops breathing, it is effective. It also works to splash water on the face. However when the case is more serious, it does not work. For example when one has drowned, it is very difficult to restore breathing. There are many cases that one has tried artificial respiration for half an hour to an hour, in vain.

(photo 31)

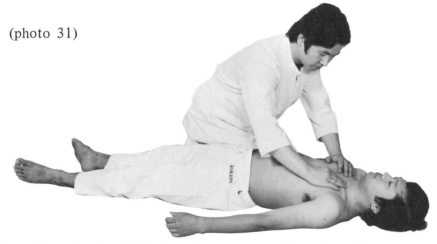

Place the patient on his back and remove any objects from his mouth. The therapist extends his four fingers and places both palms gently on the patient's chest above the nipples (phto 31). Slide both palms down the chest as if stroking in a circle. Put the two palms together under the solar plexus as if stroking in a circle (photo 32). Put the two palms together under the solar plexus (photo 33)

and press in a sudden movement toward the face (photo 34). The therapist passes his hands over the patient in a curve in order to open the patient's capillaries and cells. As shown in photo 34, do not press down on the solar plexus. It is no use. Relax the palms completely and push them toward the

(photo 32)

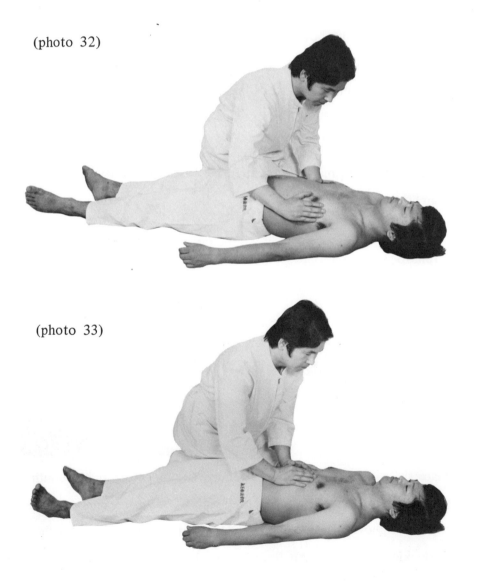

(photo 33)

face. Naturally the palms stop at the solar plexus and the breath will come out of the patient. You may practise pushing on a carpet. If you put strength in your hands and push, your hands will slip on the surface. If you relax your hands completely and push them, your skin moves slightly around the muscles and the hands naturally stop. You must practice this movement well.

(photo 34)

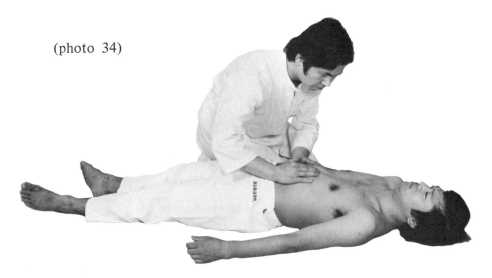

20. Melancholia

Nowadays there are many people who are melancholic or have nervous-breakdowns. It is due to the pressure from school work, jobs, and human relationships. People consume too much Ki and cannot recover. There are cases that psychosomatic medicine can solve those problems by looking into the unconscious. However there are many cases that psycosomatic medicine cannot help.

When I was young I practiced a lot of zazen or sitting meditation. I sat for at least three days and nights without a break. Of course I slept while sitting, but I never went to bed. In practising zazen, my teacher gave me a question of MU or nothingness. While thinking about the question, everything in the world started to look like nothing. When a train came toward me, the train was nothing so I started to walk toward the coming train. Fortunately I realized the danger at the last moment and escaped. When I was on a cliff and looked down, everything was nothing. I felt like I could walk down the cliff to the flowers below. If I really started to walk down, I would have died. I always realized the danger at the last moment but gradually I could not believe my perceptions. It seemed like everything was like a dream. In a cinema theatre, when everyhody else was laughing, I did not feel amused. When everybody else was happy, I did not feel anything. Gradally I did not like to meet others and stayed in my room and sat in zazen. I thought if I could be enlightened, everything would be solved but the enlightenment did not come. Even the blue sky looked grey.

One day I read a book written by a zen master and noticed that I was in zenbyo or zen illness. This kind of problem cannot be solved by psychosomatic medicine or psychology. There are people who sit in zazen for a few hours every day. This much is no problem. They will not fall ill. But many zen students who practice seriously may commit suicide because of this problem. I finally entered into the misogi training during which one breathes out completely and could come out of this illness. But I still remember the suffering I had through this period. That is why I can understand the sufferings of the people who have melancholia or a nervous breakdown. These problems are due to lack of Ki.

While awake human being consumes Ki. One must supply Ki during sleep. When one is deep asleep, the brain waves are calm and there is no obstacle to the entry of the Ki of the universe. All of the capillaries and body cells are open and relaxes so the Ki of the universe enters the body in exchange for the old Ki. It is like opening the window to change the stale air. While asleep the Ki of the universe flows into the body, so in the morning one is fresh and vigorous. When one has a problem, one cannot sleep well. The same thing happens when one studies too much and does not sleep enough. Because of lack of Ki, even in the daytime one's mind is not clear. In the night one cannot sleep well. Repeating this process one lacks Ki. When one's neck and shoulders are stiff, he cannot sleep well. During shallow sleep, the brain waves are disturbed and the entry of the Ki of the universe is hindered. If one uses the sleeping pills, the pills does not open the cells but puts the body cells in a stupor. So the Ki of the universe does not enter the cells. So one becomes deficient in Ki. To cure this lack of Ki, first do Kiatsu on lines A, B, and C of the neck so that one can move the neck freely in all directions. Next do Kiatsu on lines A and B of the back so that the nerves of the spinal cord awaken. Then send Ki into the brain through line F of the head. In this way one can sleep well that night. By repeating this, one will naturally supply a lot of Ki and the melancholia and the nervous disorder will be cured. At the same time you must teach him the principles of positive and negative and how to think in a positive way. At first one will have difficulty but by persevering, one can think positively. When both mind and body are positive, one can have a lot of Ki. It is not necessary to pull out the secrets from the unconscious. When the mind and body can turn everything positive, the past experiences do not bother him at all. Also one must practice Ki breathing in order to receive a supply of the Ki of the universe. A human being who knows his weakness can be very strong once he overcomes his weaknesses. It is useless to complain that one has a weak mind and body. It is a good chance for him to learn how to overcome his weakness.

PART TWO

Ki Exercises for Health

When one's Ki is lacking, in other words, when one is already ill or injured, we must supply Ki and activate the life power. However if the patient repeats the same mistakes in his daily life, he will have the same problems again. After curing the patient, the therapist must lead the patient so that he will not have the same problem again. Even a healthy person should learn how to live correctly so that he will not fall into problems. Just like it's better to take precautions against fire than to try to extinguish it after the fire has happend.

The nature of water is originally clean. Only when there are impurities, do we call it muddy water. A human being is originally healthy if the life power functions normally. However, most people interrupt the interchange of their own Ki and the Ki of the universe and weaken their life power. Then they think it natural that they fall ill sometimes. One must first change his ideas. "The nature of the human being is originally healthy, except when he creates reasons to fall ill".

We live in a complicated modern world suffering from the stress and the noise and have various problems to one degree or another. We often get nervous and irritated without even knowing it. When one is irritated, the blood circulation is hindered and the life power decreases and results in various diseases.

There is a physical reason for the cause of disease such as when one lives in the city and works in an office and does not get enough physical exercise. Furthermore if one always does the same exercise or uses only a part of one's body, one is apt to have problems. Occupational diseases are good examples.

I established these Four Basic Principles to Unify Mind and Body.

1. Keep the mind calm at the one point in the lower abdomen.
2. Relax completely.
3. Keep the weight of every part of the body at its lowest part.

4. Extend Ki.

The first and fourth principles are principles of the mind. The second and third are the principles of the body. If one lives in accordance with those four principles, one continuously keeps unification of mind and body. Thus the Ki of the universe interchanges with one's own Ki, and the life power is manifested at its maximum. The nature of man is to be healthy. But we all have bad habits that we've had for a long time and cannot get rid of. Though we understand with our brain, our bodies do not follow. We tend to disturb the unification of mind and body during movement.

Recently, lack of exercise has been shown to be unhealthy and many methods of exercise have been recommended. However, exercises without the correct principles do not necessarily promote health. If one continues exercises which are not in accordance with the correct principles, the body is distorted and the result can be the same as with the occupational diseases. I would now like to introduce the Ki Exercises for Health which can be done by everyone from small children to elderly people without much trouble.

1. Twisting the trunk by swinging the arms

Stand with your legs comfortably apart and swing both arms to the left with the count of 1 and 2 so that the trunk is twisted twice and the right side of the trunk is stretched. With the count of 3 and 4 do the same on the right side. Repeat this four times.

It is important to swing the arms to each side twice. If you swing to the left only once and then swing to the right, you easily lose your unification of mind and body. If you swing only once and stop when the trunk is twisted, you will easily lose balance if someone pushes your right shoulder to the left. But if you swing twice to the left and stop when the trunk is twisted, you

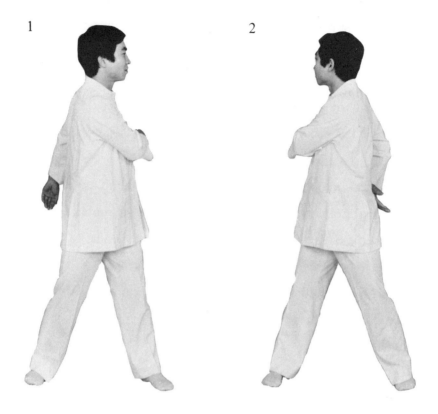

will be very stable even if someone pushes your right shoulder to the left. This means that you can keep the unification of mind and body if you swing twice. Why is there such a difference? No one noticed the big difference before. I discovered it because I know the principles of mind and body unification. We can see the body but cannot see the mind. That is why we only live physically, forgetting the existence of the mind. When we do exercises, we consider only the movement of the body and forget to exercise the mind. However, the reality is that the mind moves the body. When we walk, our mind walks using our legs. We say we walk with our legs, we do not say our legs walk. We taste food with our tongue , we do not say our tongue tastes food. The mind moves and the body follows. This is the unification of mind and body and the original great power can be manifested. If one swings his arms to each side only once, the upper body and the arms move to the side but the mind tends to be late. In other words, the direction of the mind and that of the body are not the same. Naturally one loses the unification of mind and body and becomes unstable. If one swings his arms twice to each side, the mind which was late the first time can catch up the second time so that the mind and body both move to the same direction. One keeps the unification of mind and body and is very stable. If you practice all sorts of exercises twice in the same movement every day, it becomes a habit and in the end, even if you do it only once on each side, you can still keep the unification of mind and body. This means that you can keep mind and body unfification in all activities of your daily life.

2. Bending the trunk to the side

Swing the right arm over the head to the left side twice so that the trunk bends toward the left. Do the same to the right. Repeat this four times.

3. Bending forward and backward.

Swing both arms backward over the shoulders twice so that the trunk is bent backward. With the count of 3 and 4 swing both arms and fingers between the legs twice so that the trunk is bent forward. Repeat this four times. When one bends backward even if someone pushes the shoulders down, he will be very stable. When he bends forward if his hips are pushed forward, he will not budge.

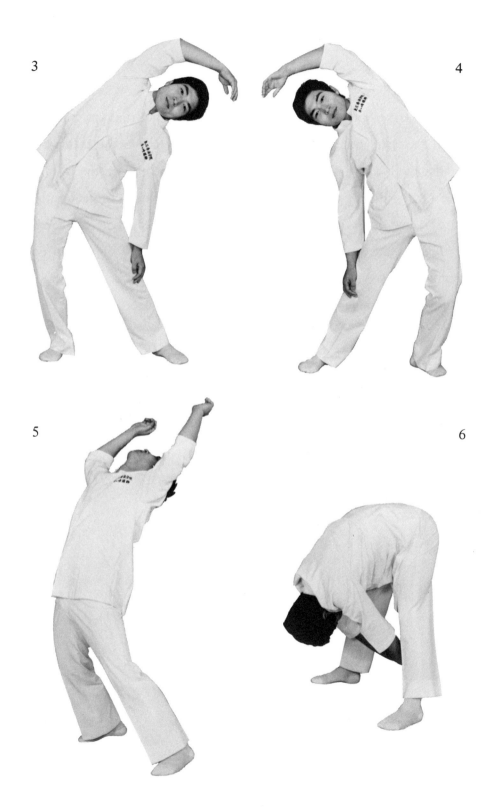

3

4

5

6

123

4. Shoulder-blade exercise

Bend the elbow and keep the hands on the same level as the shoulders. Swing the left elbow backward vigorously twice. The trunk naturally twists toward the left. The movement of the left elbow presses the D line behind the shoulder-blade and takes away the stiffness there. With the count of 3 and 4 try it with the right elbow. Repeat this four times. In the position of photo 7, one can be tested not only by being pushed at the shoulders but both elbows are so stable that they cannot be lifted or pushed down. People who play baseball or golf tend to have stiffness in the shoulder-blades. It is advisable that they make sure to do this exercise before playing.

7   8

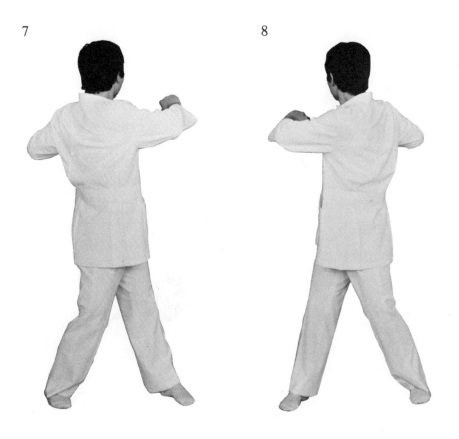

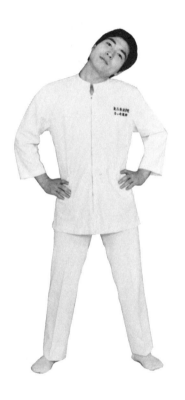
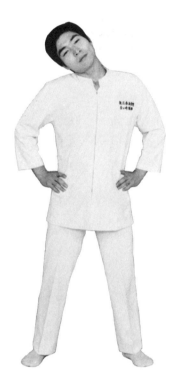

5. Bending the neck to the side

Put both hands on the hips and bend the neck to the left twice with the count of 1 and 2. Bend the neck twice to the right with the count of 3 and 4. Repeat this four times. If you bend the neck only once on each side, you will be unstable and cannot stretch the neck well. By bending the neck to the side twice from an erect position, you can stretch the neck well. Furthermore you will be very stable even if pushed from the side.

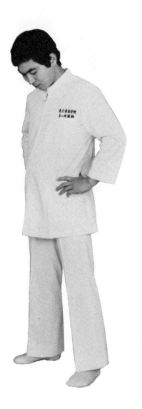 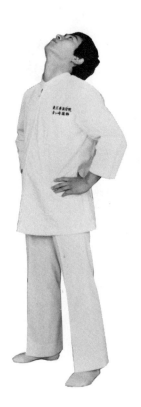

6. Bending the neck forward and backward

Starting from an erect position, bend the neck forward twice counting 1 and 2. With count of 3 and 4, bend backward. Repeat this four times. This exercise not only stretches the neck but also relaxes the back of the head.

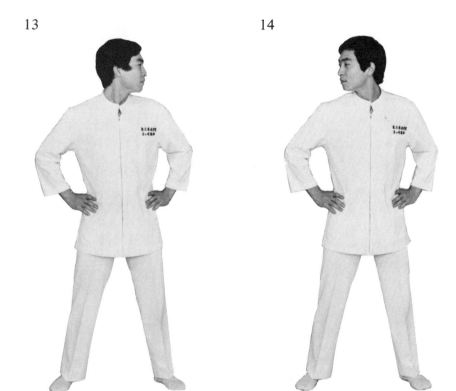

7. Turning the head to the side.

With the count of 1 and 2, turn the head twice to the left and with the count of 3 and 4, turn it twice to the right. Repeat this four times.

All these neck exercises relax the neck and head and prevent headaches and stiff shoulders.

15 16

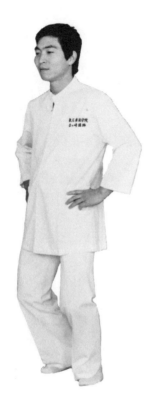
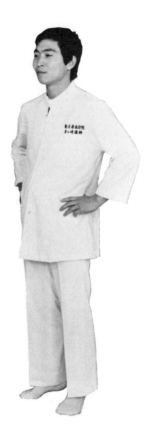

8. Knee exercises

With the count of 1 and 2, bend the knees twice keeping the hands on the hips and the upper body erect and calm. With the count of 3 and 4 lift the heels twice and come down. Repeat this four times. In the position of photo 15, even if someone tries to push you down by putting his hands on your hips and pushes down, you will not budge. But if you bend your knees only once and stop, you will be pushed down.

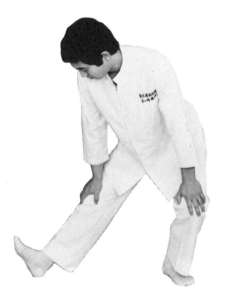
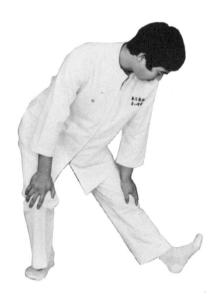

9. Stretching the knees

Stand with legs comfortably apart and put your hands on the knees. With the count of 1 and 2, stretch the right knee by bending the left knee. Lift the right toes to stretch the knee. Stretch the right knee twice helping with the right hands. With the count of 3 and 4, stretch the left knee in the same manner. Repeat this four times. In the position of photo 17, the stretched right leg is so heavy that the foot cannot be lifted by someone else. But if you stretch it only once, your right foot will easily be lifted.

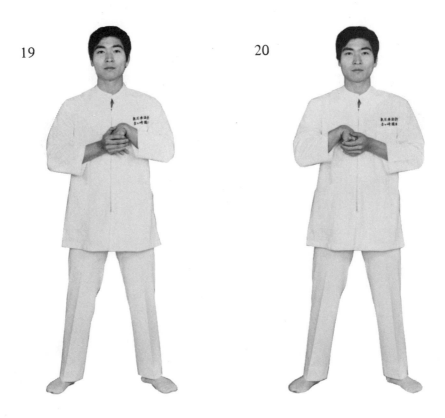

19   20

10 Wrist bending exercise (1)

Bend the left wrist and put the right palm on the back of the left hand. With the count of 1, 2, 3, 4, push the left hand with the right palm four times so that the back of the left hand is stretched. Try the same with the other side. Repeat this twice. When you bend the wrist, do not put strength and force it to bend. If you put strength, all the body cells contract and do not stretch. Do it comfortably so that you have a nice feeling. When you relax, the muscles stretch well.

In the position of photo 19 if someone tries to push your wrist further, if you relax completely, you will not feel any pain. However if you try to force your wrist to bend and someone else applies more pressure, you will feel tremendous pain.

21 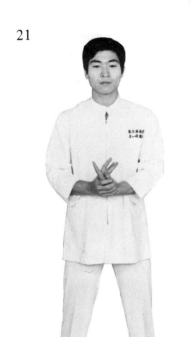 22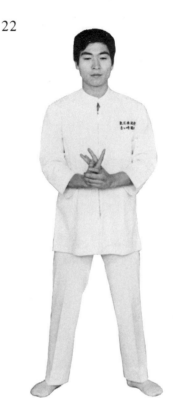

11 Wrist bending exercise (2)

Put your left hand in front of you with palm up and bend the little finger side upward. Put your right palm on the back of the left hand. With the count of 1, 2, 3, 4, bring both hands down so that the right hand naturally bends the left wrist toward the little finger. Try the same with the other side. Repeat this twice. Do not force the wrist to bend. It will only make the wrist weak. It is very important to stretch the muscles comfortably and easily.

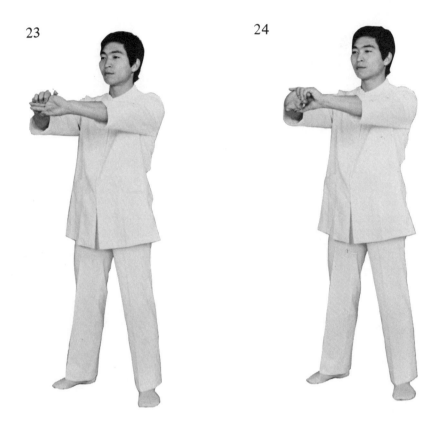

23   24

12. Wrist stretching exercise

Put your left hand in front of you with the little finger side up and the palm facing forward. Hold the left hand from above with your right hand. With the count of 1, 2, 3, 4, push both hands forward so that the little finger side of the left hand is stretched four times. Do the same with the other side. Repeat this twice. In the position of photo 23, your two hands will not be pushed back even if someone tries to push them back toward you. But if you use force to stretch muscles and put strength, you will be easily push back.

25 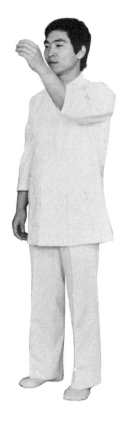 26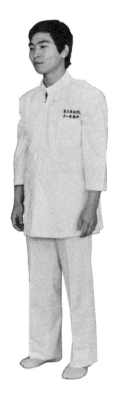

13. Arm swinging exercise

Put your right arm forward. (photo 25) Relax your arm completely and let your right arm fall down (photo 26). The right elbow will naturally bend a little. With the count of 1, let your right arm fall down and the momentum will make the arm go up in a circle naturally (photo 27). Swing your arm like this four times with the count of 1,2,3,4. Do the same with the left arm. Repeat this twice. The universe moves with rhythm. The blowing wind, the flowing river, everything moves with rhythm. Without rhythm, there is no power. There is a rhythm for swinging the arm. When it falls down, it gets quicker and when it goes up, naturally it slow down. If the first downward

27

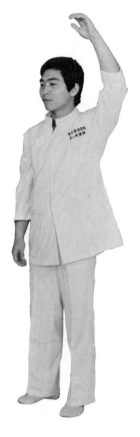

motion is strong, the second down swing becomes naturally powerful. But
if you put strength while the arm is going up, you will have no power when
the arm comes down. However, many people put strength when the arm
goes up, and want to bring the arm down strongly. This unreasonable movement damages the shoulders or elbow. If one knows this principle, one will
never hurt the shoulders or elbows when playing baseball, tennis, or golf.
One can play very well with a lot of power,. In the position of figure 26, you
will be very stable if somebody tries to pull your hand down or push it up
toward the shoulder. If you put strength and bring down your arm, you
will easily be unbalanced when somebody pulls or pushes your hand. One
must make a habit of swinging the arm with a natural rhythm.

28   29

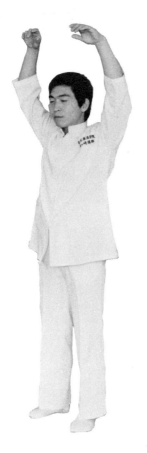   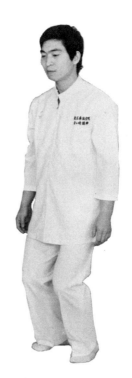

14. Swinging both arms

Swing both arms with the count of 1, 2, 3, and 4. Next with the count of
1, 2, 3, and 4, swing both arms in the opposite direction. Repeat this twice.
Next try the same exercise while bending and strethcing the knees, using the
same rhythm. Do this four times to the front and four times to the back.
Repeat this twice. This exercise will improve the blood circulation and rel-
laxation of the shoulders, arms , and legs.

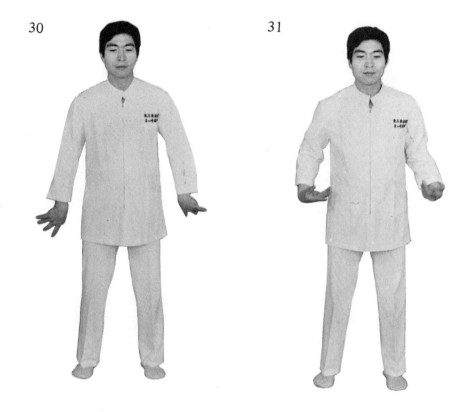

30   31

15. Wrist shaking exercise

Stand naturally keeping one point. The feet are side by side and spaced a natural distance with the arms hanging down naturally. Shake the finger-tips as quickly as possible with the one point as the center so that the vibration goes to every part of the body. In this way you can disperse all the stiffness of the body. If you use strength, you will not be able to shake quickly. By shaking the hands as quickly as possible, you can relax. Try this exercise as the finishing exercise.

I have explained 15 exercises in all. It will take you about three minutes. Even the busiest person in the world can find three minutes' spare time a day. You can do it at home or in the office. All the exercises are done with a four beat rhythm. You can do them to music with four beat time. Try them and enjoy them.

16. Leg stretching exercises

The preceding exercises were all done in the standing position. You can even do them in the park. They can be done by many people together. Now I explain the stretching exercises for the legs which are done in a sitting position.

32   33

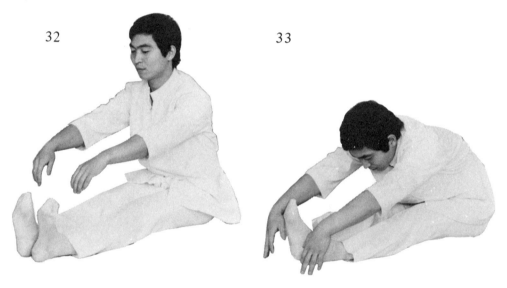

(1) Stretch your legs forward with the heels out. Going over the feet try to touch the floor with your fingertips. Do this five times with the count of five. Repeat this twice. At first, most people will hardly be able to touch the toes. Do not force yourself. Try it every day with a relaxed rhythm. Little by little the muscles and tendons in the back of the leges will stretch and you will be able to touch the floor by going over the feet. This exercise stretches the line C of the leg. Make sure your heels are pushed out to the front.

34

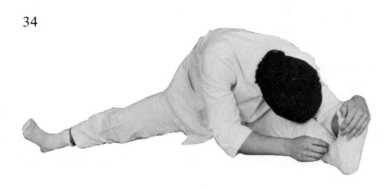

35

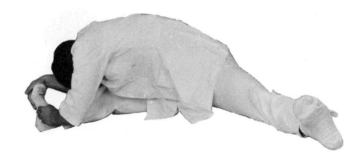

(2) Spread your legs apart as much as possible. Hold the left toes with your left hand and push out the left heel. Try to touch the left leg with your chest and head (photo 34). This is done with five counts. This exercise stretches the line F of the leg. Next stretch the right leg in the same way (photo 35). Repeat this twice. After stretching the left leg, spread it more with the left hand. You will be able to open it more because the tendon stretches. Always open a little more after each stretching. You will come to find that you can spread your legs much more than before.

36

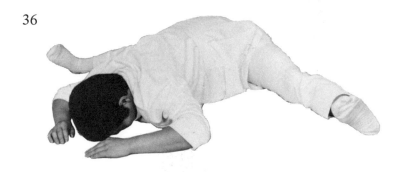

37

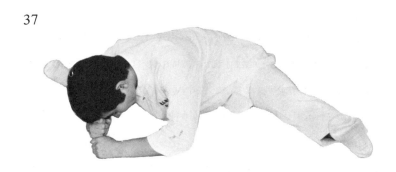

(3) When the legs are well stread, bend your upper body forward so that the head touches the floor. Try this five times keeping a good rhythm.

Repeat this twice. Most people will not succeed in touching the floor with the head. If this is the case, then place both fists, one over another, on the floor in front of you and try to touch them with your head (photo 37). By doing this exercise with a relaxed rhythm, soon you will be able to touch the floor with the head. One must continue with patience. This exercise stretches the line G of the legs.

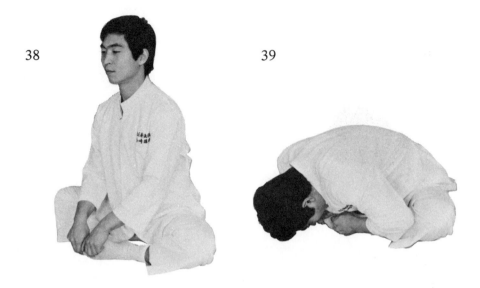

38   39

(4)   Bend your knees and put both soles together in front of you. If the
knees are up in the air, try to bring them down to the floor. (photo 38) Try
this with a relaxed rhythm several times. Draw both feet close to the stomach
and bend your upper body forward so that the head touches the floor going
over the feet (photo 39). Do this counting from 1 to 5. Repeat this twice.
This exercise stretches the line G of the leg. When the line G is stiff, the
knees will not go down to the floor. This exercise also stretches the lower
back. If the lower back is stiff, it can cause a hernia of the vertebrae.

(5)   Sit on your knees. Place your big toes one over another. Lay back-
wards putting your upper body on the floor. Stretch both arms back with

40

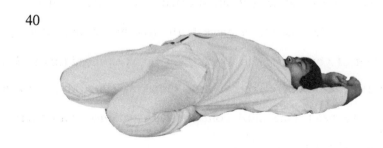

the palms up stretching the upper body well.

This exercise stretches not only the thighs but also the lower stomach. It will improve the conditions of the intestines, making it good for chronic digestive problems.

17. Rolling exercise

Sit down with your legs crossed. (photo 41). On the count of 1, roll backward (photo 42), and at the count of 2, return to the sitting posture (photo 43) When you return, you must remain in that position. At this time another person will try to push the shoulders backward. If you fall back, you did not keep your mind and body unified. In photo 42 the mind and body go backward together so that the legs go up easily and in photo 43 both the mind and body must go forward together. Then you will be very stable even if another person pushes you. Most people leave their minds behind when

41   42

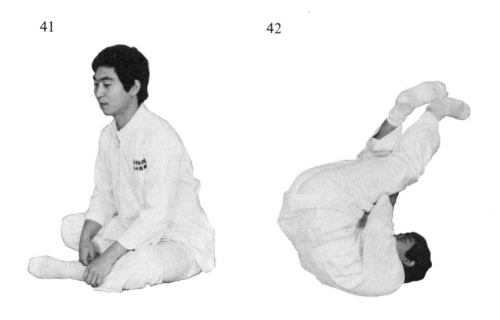

43

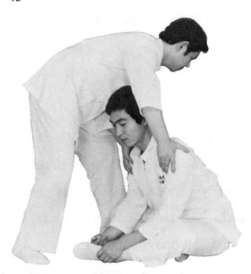

their bodies return forward. So they are very weak. One must extend Ki forward when the body comes forward. In this exercise the entire spine will make contact with the floor. So it is similar to the floor massaging the back. But one must do it with unification of mind and body. When a tank is full of gas, a little spark can cause a big explosion. When a person unifies his mind and body, his body is full of Ki, and a little stimulation will start the Ki extending. So the life power is greatly enhanced. By doing this exercise with the mind and body unified, the Ki extends through the back. The messages from the brain pass through the spinal column and reach the whole body. So when the Ki is activated there, the life power is activated throughout the body. It is the best Ki exercises for health.

A human being is very soft when he is a baby. But as he grows up, he becomes stiffer and when he is completely stiff, he is dead. A stiff body means that you are nearing death. On the contrary if the body gets softer, then you are getting younger. Do not be discouraged even if your body is stiff now. By doing these exercises every day in a relaxed manner and without force, your body will gradually become soft. The whole group of standing and sitting exercises will take only five minutes. No matter how busy you are, you can spare five minutes a day. If you want to keep healthy, you must keep your mind and body flexible. But do not forget that no one else can take care of you. You must take care of yourself.

PART THREE

Medical Lecture

(by Dr. Kanemizu Ariizumi)

Chapter $\boxed{1}$ Fundamentals of Cure

Sickness is the opposite of good health. Sickness means the state of continuing life with abnormal physiology. In other words, health means to live normally and sickness means to live abnormally. But the borderline between normal and abnormal life is difficult to define since it changes according to the occasions and circumstances. We could say there is a sphere of being normal and when one is out of this sphere, he is considered to be ill.

Medically, life means the metabolism of matter, energy, and form. In the cell body health means high metabolism and sickness means low metabolism. A cell body takes in the nutrients, creates the vital power with the help of enzymes and oxygen, and gives out waste materials. The origin of vital power can be scientifically analyzed as heat, light, electricity, etc. The scientists can also clearify the synthesis and decomposition of the chemical procedures performed in the human body. However, science has not determined who is doing all these chemical processes and what kind of power is creating the vital power from all the chemical reactions. This original power is called mind power. Naturally the mind can strengthen the vital power. There is a limit for the physical power but no limit to the mental power. Then what is the origin of the physical and mental power? Each religion and philosophy gives many different names but in Japan this is normally called Ki. The origin of everything is Ki. The human being is also born from Ki and cannot live without Ki. When we do not have enough Ki, the vital power is low and results in illness. The fundamentals of cure is to activate the curing power which human beings originally have. Living is an interchange between the Ki of the universe and the individual Ki in the human body. When this interchange is high, one is vigorous. When one extends Ki, naturally new Ki from the universe comes into the body, resulting in a good interchange of Ki. When the body is full of Ki, the curing power works at its maximum.

A sick person recovers very quickly if he forgets about his illness. But it is very difficult to forget about it. Many people worry about it and make their minds disturbed. When the mind is not stable, the Ki of the universe does not come in, so the body becomes weaker. If one wants to recover from illness, he must first keep his mind calm. However, many people disturb their minds wanting to recover quickly. It is like someone walking to the west thinking he wants to go to the east. So it is very important to calm the mind when one is ill.

The curing methods can be classified as follows.

1. Giving Ki directly

Using this method a person gives Ki directly to the patient by being near as a positive influence. Just like heat flows from a warm place to a cold place, strong Ki flows to weaker Ki. The Ki of the stronger person flows to the sick person. The sick person is naturally assimilated by the mind of the stronger person and the sick person's Ki increases. If a person of strong Ki stays with a sick person, the sick person can recover. However, the stronger person who gives Ki must always unify his mind and body and have a good interchange of Ki with the universe so that he gets a good supply of Ki from the universe. Otherwise the stronger person can become ill.

2. Kiatsu Ryoho

Kiatsu Ryoho was created by Master Koichi Tohei. It is a method of pouring Ki to the diseased part of the patient from the fingertips. A sick person's diseased part especially lacks life force and the vital power is low. The priming Ki from the therapist to the diseased part will stimulate the life power of the sick person. Then the blood circulation is improved and the oxygen and nutrients in the blood stream are well-absorbed by the body cell. The quantity of the leucocytes which are functional increases. Even modern medicine's cure is fundamentally to take away the harmful things and activate the natural healing powers of the patient. There are many methods in modern medicine, operation, medications, injections, physical therapy, etc. But they often cause after-effects. Doctors must always consider if the method is worth doing in spite of the ill side effects.

3. Remote cure

This method is better understood from a philosophical or religious perspective rather than medical theory. A person of strong Ki uses his will power in order to activate the Ki and the vital powers of the sick person, even at a distance.

4. Breathing method

The best way to cure a disease by oneself is by using the breathing method. The breath of a healthy person is calm and strong. An unhealthy person always breathes short and rough. A human being can live without eating for several weeks but cannot stop breathing even for several minutes. That is why breathing is very important for the cure. Breathing deeply with mind and body unified gives the following effects;

It gives abundant oxygen to the body cell, removes the carbonic acid gas and other waste matters smoothly, relaxes the body, and calms the mind.

The interbrain at the center of the autonomic nervous system controls the breathing, blood circulation, digestion, absorption, secretion, etc. Emotions and thinking are also performed in the interbrain, so that when one worries or is anxious, immediately the heart starts beating quickly and the breathing shortens. Sometimes the face even becomes white. The face becomes white because the capillary vessels contract with the tension of the autonomic nervous system. When the capillary vessels contract, blood circulation is blocked. In addition, the abnormal secretion of harmones causes an abnormal increase of sugar in the blood. This excess of sugar oxidizes in the blood. The normal blood is week alkaline and the leucocytes are highly functional, but if the blood is acid, the leucocytes cannot work well. So breathing with mind and body unified relaxes the autonomic nervous system and prevents the above ill effects.

5. Sleep cure

Next to Ki breathing, sleeping is the most effective method to cure disease. One can absorb the vital power from the Ki of the universe while sleeping. When one relaxes completely, keeping his mind very calm, and letting himself completely to the universe, the Ki of the universe pours into his body. A healthy person can sleep well and absorbs the Ki of the universe. An unhealthy person sleeps badly and cannot absorb the Ki of the universe so that he becomes more and more unhealthy. One must learn how to sleep well.

Chapter 2 How to Maintain Health

1. The life force

Before thinking about health, one should understand what life is. Then what is life? To understand this, he must get rid of all his preconceptions and see the universe as it is. Then he will understand that one's life flows with the movement of the universe. One will understand that the Ki of the universe is the same Ki which maintains one's life. One can understand that his life is a part of the universe, not as a theory, but as a fact. So our lives cannot exist apart from the Ki of the universe. In other words, we live under the control of the universe and our health methods must follow the principles of the universe.

The natural life is a relaxed life. But it is very difficult to relax. If you really want to relax, you must first unify your mind and body. This is the best way of life and follows the principles of the universe. To maintain health, you must know and follow the principles of the universe. Also, the human body has an adaptability to the environment. One can promote health by increasing this adaptability. To summarize, through the unification of mind and body the vital power of the Ki of the universe is absorbed. And in order to guide this life power to all the parts of the body, one must exercise adaptability.

2. An effect of mind and body unification.

In November 1972 we took video photos of the stomach of Master Koichi Tohei. He can freely control his pulse rate. I first asked him to increase his pulse. He imagined the state of being angry and his pulse rose to 98 beats per minute. When his pulse quickened his stomach stopped digestive movements. Next I asked him to unify his mind and body. The pulse rate slowed to 60 per minute and the stomach began functioning again. Naturally when the stomach works well, gastric juices flow properly and the food in the stomach can be digested well. All the digestive system is controlled by the same nervous system so that all the organs and glands work well and the secretion levels are correct. At this time the liver, the spleen, kidneys, and other related organs also function well .

From this experiment we can understand that anger gives a shock to the body through the nervous system, which is called stress. As a result the function of the digestive system becomes abnormally low. It is easy to get angry, sad, or afraid, but it is very difficult to return to calmness. Most people believe their minds cannot move so easily. Those people do not know how to control their own minds. One reason why it is very difficult to control the mind is because of the problems of the unconscious mind. However, by learning unification of mind and body, all the organs function well so the fundamentals of cure and the fundamentals of maintenance of health are exactly one.

3. How to promote the life power.

Health means to absorb enough vital power from the environment and use this vital power in the whole body. Investigating this question more in detail, the following points surface:

1. How is this vital power used in the human body?

2. What is the source of the vital power?

3. How is the vital power absorbed?

The first point is very important but many people do not pay attention to it because it is not visible to the eye. All the organs and the body cells are working to change nutrition, air, and sunshine into the vital power. One must not interfere with this process. When one unifies his mind and body, all the organs function well. If one disturbs his mind, this function is interrupted, and the vital power decreases. The waste matters are not discharged well so that they remain in the body and are harmful to the body cells. Naturally when the body cells are damaged, the organs do not function well so that the health is in turn damaged. Disturbances of the mind, such as anger, fear or sorrow separate mind and body and the health decreases.

Since second and third points are interrelated they are explained together. The sources of the vital power are the following:

Air

The air is very important for the vital power. Food is oxidized and changed into ATP. When this ATP is decomposed to ADP and phosphoric acid, energy is released. This energy is the source of the vital power. This ATP increases when oxygen increases. Air is composed of the following gases.

Oxygen	20.99%
Nitrogen	78,03%
Carbonic dioxide	0.03%
Argon	0.94%
Hydrogen	0.01%

There are also traces of neon, helium, krypton, xenon, etc.

This is the composition of clean air and normally various bacteria and dust are also found in air. The oxygen in the air is most important for the vital power. The nitrogen is also important in the sense that it dilutes the oxygen so that we human beings can breathe well. Carbonic acid gas, ammonia, nitric acid and sulphuric acid are harmful to the health. It is important to be in fresh air. Breathing is principally done by the lung but the skin also breathes. One must be careful for the circulation of air on the skin surface.

Breathing means to take in oxygen and push out the carbon dioxide. Outside breathing or lung breathing means to take in air into the lungs and push out the carbon dioxide from the lungs. Internal breathing or tissue breathing means to take the oxygen from the lungs to the capillaries and give the tissues oxygen and carries the carbon dioxide from the tissue to the lungs.

Without oxygen the nutrients cannot be converted into energy. So when the body is full of oxygen, the life power is fully activated. After the energy is released, the carbon dioxide and waste matters are formed and they must be carried to the lung in the blood stream and pushed out by exhaling. If carbon dioxide is accumulated in the body, assimilation of the nutrients slows and the maintenance of life becomes more difficult. Blood in the arteries is red with much oxygen and the blood in the veins is dark with waste matters and carbon dioxide. So it is very important to exhale the carbon dioxide. The composition of the expiration is the following:

Oxygen   16.4%

Carbon dioxide   4.1% (2.5 to 4.6%)

Nitrogen   79.5%

When fresh air is breathed, the oxygen rate goes down from 20% to 16% and carbon dioxide increases from 0.03% to 4%. The breathing capacity of a Japanese adult is as follows:

Man   3000 to 4000 cc

Woman   2500 to 3500 cc

A normal breath is 500 cc.

The best way to increase the vital power is to take in maximum amount of oxygen by good breathing. The hemoglobin in the blood takes in the oxygen from the lung cell and carries the oxygen to the body tissues. The oxygen is given to the tissue and the carbon dioxide is taken by the capillaries. It is very important to open every capillary so that the blood runs smoothly. To do this one must relax his mind and body. That means when one unifies his mind and body, the capillary vessels open and the circulation of blood is good. Therefore, it is very important to master unification of mind and body to do Ki breathing. The Ki breathing is long and calm so that the partial pressure of oxygen in the lungs is high, giving more oxygen to the blood.

Even though you may understand that Ki breathing is the best method to activate the life power, unless you actually practice it, it is useless. You must try it yourself. There are several effects you can get from Ki breathing.

a) Improving the liver's function.

The liver is a vital organ for the maintenance of life.

Its functions are:

1) decomposing the nutrition into the vital energy and storing nutrition.
2) neutralizing the poisonous products which are taken into the body or produced in the body.
3) secreting bile
4) producing the anti-bodies which guard against bacteria
5) controlling the quantity of the blood circulating
6) controlling metabolism of vitamins
7) controlling hormones

The liver has many functions so it needs a lot of the vital energy. Therefore the liver contains a lot of blood and is full of capillary vessels.

Naturally it consumes a lot of oxygen. Evidently by increasing the oxygen in the blood by the Ki breathing, the functions of liver improve. These are some examples:

1) In Hawaii a middle-aged man was going to hospital for over a year for liver problems. After continuing Ki breathing an hour every day for three months, his liver was completely cured.

2) There was a Ki breathing session of five days, one hour each day. Attending was a man of 79 who had been suffering from allergic sinusitis. He had been going to various doctors, in vain. After three days his nose was all right and he has never had problems since then. This must be because his liver was improved.

3) A man of 65 had high blood pressure and a heart problem. So he was taking a lot of medication. However he started Ki breathing thirty minutes every morning and evening and after two months his illnesses were cured. Also his athlete's foot which had been with him for thirty years vanished. This is also due to the enforced liver function.

4) With Ki breathing, one can return to a normal state much quicker after drinking alcohol. It is also partly due to the enforced liver function.

b) Improving the kidney function.

The liver and the kidneys are very closely related. The liver neutralizes the poisonous products and the kidneys eliminate the waste matters. In blood waste matters and nurishment are mixed together.

When the liver does not decompose the waste matters sufficiently or neutralize the poisonous products, the kidneys must overwork and get tired. That will lead to kidney problems and finally the whole body swells or protein is thrown out in the urine. In modern medicine the kidney problems are treated together with liver. Besides, the kidneys are also influenced by the mind so it is very important to calm the mind. The kidneys are consisted of many capillary vessels. When one does Ki breathing and unifies his mind and body, the mind is calm and the capillary vessels open so that blood full of oxygen can pass. Naturally the kidneys function well and all the waste matters in the body are eliminated in urine. So it improves all the other organs and retards senility.

c) Improving the brain

The brain is the heaviest organ requiring a lot of blood circulation. If the brain cells lack in oxygen for three minutes, they will die. The oxygen is the dire necessity for the brain. Naturally abundant oxygen will improve the brain function.

d) Improving the function of stomach and intestines.

This is already explained in the previous chapter.

e) Effect on the heart and the lungs

The heart and the lungs are the main organs which function in the Ki breathing. Naturally their function is improved.

f) Help against cancer

Modern medicine and the governments of most countries are very interested in the research of cancer and its cure. Radiation can be used to destroy the cancer cells and when there is abundant oxygen around the cancer cell, the effectiveness of the cure is high. The normal cells around the cancer cells are activated by oxygen and have strong resistance against the cancer cell.

Naturally the Ki breathing must help to hinder the growth of cancer.

Food

1) The correct attitude toward eating

Food is necessary for the maintenance of life. To eat means to take in the vital power of the food in the human body. It is very well explained in "Ki in Daily Life" written by Master Koichi Tohei. He explains that the life of the food exists with the human life and that one must take a meal with gratitude. This attitude means that one is relaxed and the mind is calm. It means one unifies his mind and body in his daily life. It is also true medically.

2) Food therapy

There is no special diet. A natural diet is best. Modern dietetics is well-developed and many discuss calories, etc. But many people forget the state of the person who takes the meal. A person's being overweight or under-weight, his amount of physical exertion, and sleeping habits affect the ability to absorb nurishments. Requirements vary with the state of the person. They also need different alimentation. It is not unnecessary to think about calories and diet but it is far more important to improve the condition of the body of he who takes the meal. There are several important points for eating:

a) Eat when you are hungry.

It is very natural that hunger is the best sauce. However many take meals because the time of the meals has come. It is better not to take meals if you are not hungry. A person with weak stomach and intestines especially must take care. Appetite normally goes together with hunger but one must be aware that he can sometimes have appetite without hunger. It is not necessary to have three meals a day. Two meals a day may suffice. The important principle is that one eats when he is hungry. Then the food tastes good and the digestive organs absorb the nurishments well. When one lacks sleep or has a big problem or anxiety, the stomach stops functioning and the appetite disappears. In that case first sleep well and then eat. If you have a problem or anxiety, you must change your mind to another thing. But it is not easy to control the mind. That is why we must practice the unification of mind and body.

b) Mastication and saliva

Everyone knows the importance of mastication but saliva is also very important to human health. Ingestion means to chew the food well, mix it with saliva, and send the food to the stomach. The longer one chews the food, the better it is digested and absorbed in the stomach and intestines.

Starch in the food is digested by the amylase in saliva into maltose. If mastication is not sufficient, the starches are not well-digested by the salvia and the digestive tract weakens. If one chews well, adequate saliva is secreted. The secretion of saliva is influenced not only by the taste of the food but also by the mind. When the mind is disturbed, the saliva secretion is inadequate. And when the mind is calm, saliva secretion is high. One can increase salivation through Ki meditations.

One of the salivary glands secretes a hormone called parotin. This hormone prevents senility, promotes the manufacture of blood, the growth of hair and the growth of cartilage. Mastication increases not only the secretion of saliva but also the hormones from the salivary glands. Good mastication is important not only for digestion but also benefits the whole body.

c) Food

Nourishment in food can be classified into the following five categories: 1. Water 2. Protein 3. Fat 4. Sugar 5. Vitamins and minerals Food and drink are very important as the source metabolism in human life. However when we take food, we take also the bacteria and other harmful things which we must be very careful to avoid. Meat especially always has some decomposition called ptomaine. If one takes a large quantity of ptomaine, it causes poisoning and is dangerous to life. When choosing meat, one must be careful to take fresh meat. However we normally do not kill an animal and eat it immediately. There is always a time after killing the animal so there is always a little ptomaine. Therefore to avoid too much rotten matter, vegetables are better than meat. It is true that vegetarians normally live longer.

Vegetables also calm and stabilize the mind. It is not meaningless that zen priests eat vegetables. Yoga people do not eat meat and live long lives. Some people think that vegetables do not give stamina but the truth is that the blood has strong bacteria destroying power when it is slightly alkaline. When the blood changes to the acid, the bacteria destroying power decreases. Vegetables make the blood more alkaline and meat makes the blood more acid. By eating more vegetables and less meat, one contracts fewer illness and can recover more quickly.

Sugar also makes the blood acid, so it is better not to consume too much sugar, either.

Fruit is also good for the health but in some places it is difficult to obtain and can be expensive. Using modern cooking methods people sometimes have a tendency to cook food with many condiments. Moderate cooking is good to promote the secretion of saliva but too much cooking particularly with condiments for satisfying the tongue can sometimes harm the body. The essence of cooking is to enhance the original and natural taste of the food. Recently natural food has become popular. It has its merit but important thing is to eat not to satisfy taste but to maintain life.

Dieticians often discuss the calories in food. It is interesting as science but in daily life only calories do not make good diet. For example, water has no calories and no nourishment but if there is not enough water in the body, the digestion and absorption of food will suffer. If 20% of the body water is lost, the life is in danger. Two thirds of a human being's weight is water. Water is always lost from the body during perspiration, exhalation, and urination. 3000 to 4000 cc of water is lost every day. It is very important to take water. Adults take enough water because they have the ability to satisfy thirst, but mothers with small babies should be careful to provide enough water. When a person learns a lot about dietetics, he might be at a loss how to satisfy all his knowledge. But a human being is born from nature and can live well naturally. When one's mind is calm, he naturally wants to eat what is necessary for him. Unification of mind and body is the natural state of a human being.

Sleep

Sleep restores fatigue and promotes good health. It is very well explained in "Ki in Daily Life" written by Master Koichi Tohei. Medically, sleep is a state that the brain is calm. The brain waves during Ki meditation and sleep are very similar. At the University of California the aura of the human body was photographed. They took kirlian photos after five minutes of Ki meditation. The aura became much larger than before, verifying that the life power was activated. After deep sleep the aura increases. Children normally sleep well but many adults cannot sleep well. It is due to the fact that their minds are disturbed in the daytime and still are not calm at night. When one tries to sleep, his effort disturbs the mind. One must learn how to unify the mind. Sometimes people take sleeping pills. When one sleeps with the help of sleeping pills, the brain cells are anaesthetized. The brain waves are not calm so one does not recover the life power. It is better not to take sleeping pills. One must learn the real method for sleeping.

Sunshine

Maintenance of life is impossible without sunshine. The sun protects our lives. Without the sun our lives could not exist on earth. We must be grateful of this fact. The sunbeams can be divided into seven colors, red, orange, yellow, green blue, indigo, and violet. Their wave lengths range from 760 mu to 400 mu. The infra-red (1,000 mu to 760 mu) and the ultra-violet (400 mu to 100 mu) are also included. Infra-red rays are also called heat rays. Ultra violet rays are also called chemical rays because they cause many chemical reactions.

a) The function of ultra-red rays to the human body.

They penetrate deep into the tissue without being absorbed in the pigment and give heat to the blood vessels.

b) Effects of ultra-violet rays on the human body.

1) They increase the red corpuscles and lymphocytes which promote the internal breathing and increase antibodies.

2) They enlarge the capillaries and decrease the blood pressure. Naturally it promotes the metabolism and increases the life power.

3) They deepen the breathing, increase the urination, accelerate the appetite, and improve the sleep.

4) They promote the manufacture and accumulation of vitamin D, and accelerate the increase of phosphorus and calcium in blood.

5) They accelerate skin breathing, perspiration, secretion of skin oils and make the skin beautiful.

6) They promote pain relief and scab formation. A wound can be cured very quickly by exposing it to the sun. It prevents keloid.

7) They kill bacteria. Ultra-violet rays are a very important function of sunbeams. They kill suppurative germs in 5 to 10 seconds, tuberculosis

germs and diphtheria germs in 10 to 20 seconds, cholera germs, typhoid germs, and dysentery germs in 10 to 50 seconds. Disinfection by the sun is very useful for health.

8) They also tan the skin.

The ultra-violet rays are stronger in higher places and in southern areas. They are also stronger in summer than in winter and strongest in the midday.

The sunshine has many effects on the human body. If one is exposed too much to direct sunshine, it can cause headache, dizziness, or weariness. A sunbath of a sick person must be conducted by a doctor. A healthy person sunbathes using this guideline: when sitting calmly in the sun, if one perspires, it is a sign of excess sunshine. One must gradually adapt himself to the sun. A person who is used to the sunshine, will not have many side-effects. It is a matter of adaptability. The sunshine also influences the nervous system, usually making the mind positive. In Japan there is a proverb that a house with a lot of sunshine does not need a doctor. One fares better to make use of the sunshine. The best method is to do Ki exercises or Ki breathing under the morning sun without clothes.

Earth

The soil of the earth has a lot of energy. Chemical wastes from factories can be decomposed and neutralized in the soil. It's a good feeling to go to the countryside, lie down on the soil and look at the sky. Walking on the soil with bare feet is also very comfortable. Soil gives energy to the human body. There are therapies making use of the soil energy. Painting mud on the skin or taking a mud bath can cure neuralgia or rheumatism. Besides this, the soil gives energy to plants which in turn gives us energy as food. They protects our lives as well as the sun does. Do not forget to make use of the benefits of soil.

Excretion

Excretion means to remove the waste materials from the body. It is done in the form of evacuation, urination, perspiration, and exhalation. Excretion does not give energy but it is necessary for good metabolism. Waste materials accumulated in the body can cause illness.

a) Evacuation

Evacuation of feces is very important to maintain good health. Constipation is a proof of inactive intestines. It means the blood circulation around the intestines is not good. This causes many symptoms in other parts of the body, headaches, stiff shoulders, dizziness, lack of appetite, insomnia, etc. The most important thing to prevent constipation is to activate the intestinal movement.

The intestines are controlled by the autonomic nerves. That means we cannot consciously control the intestines. However the mental stress strains the pneumogastric nerves which slackens the movement of the intestines. So stress causes constipation. Therefore it is very important to calm the mind or unify mind and body. When Master Tohei's stomach and intestines were X-rayed in the state of mind and body unification, they were active. He imagines washing the intestines when evacuating feces. In this way he promotes evacuation. This includes very important questions. It is possible to use the unconscious mind by the unification of mind and body in order to control the sympathetic nerves so that they activate the intestines. Doctors suggest going to toilet regularly at a fixed time. By forming a conditioned reflex, one can control the central nervous system to activate the intestines. Kiatsu on the belly directly activates the intestines. It activates not only intestines but also all the internal organs in the belly. It is very good for the health to do Kiatsu on your own belly before going to sleep. We are very conscious of the muscular fatigue of arms and legs but we do not easily notice the fatigue of internal organs.

Urination

When urination is normal, people do not think of it. However, if urination is blocked, urea and uric acid increase in the blood and cause urine poisoning. Urine is produced by filtering the waste materials in the blood in the kidneys. When the kidneys have problems, it shows in the urine. Besides, the liver, the pancreas, and the heart also change the urine. The kidneys are controlled by the autonomic nerves and hormones. It is important to unify the mind and body so that the mind is always calm and without stress.

Chapter 3 How to Strengthen the Resistance to Disease

Life is an adaptation to the change of environments, specially change in climate, food, noise, bacteria, etc. A person of small adaptability can fall ill easily. It is, therefore, very important to improve the resistance, or adaptability to the change of environment. One can increase resistance little by little. For example, one may easily get tired after two kilometers' walk on the first day. But if one increases the distance little by little every day, he can easily walk five or ten kilometers without fatigue. It is because a resistance was formed to the walking exercises. But when one trains resistance, he should be careful not to increase the exercise too quickly. Overwork can consume the body and causes sickness. It is very important to increase the training gradually.

Another important point is to train with mind and body unified. Master Tohei said, "When we unify our mind and body and become one with the universe, we can manifest our great power which is originally ours." All the human organs are controlled by the nerves. When a strong Ki comes through the nerves, the nerves make the organs work very strongly. Training with the mind and body unified provides maximum effects. The unification of mind and body is most important to increase resistance.

1. Improving the resistance of skin

The skin is covering the human body and touches the environments. It is like a sentry line of the army. When the sentinel is not functioning well, the enemy can penetrate and attack the army. When the resistance of the skin decreases, the bacteria can penetrate and cause illness. By increasing the resistance of the skin, one can prevent many diseases.

Many capillaries run on the skin. Nerves also run with the capillaries. The nerves control the function of the skin. The nerves enlarge or contract the capillary vessels and adjust to the temperature. The nerves also control the tactile sense, the sense of heat, the sense of cold, the sense of pain, and perspiration. If the skin does not adjust to the change of temperature, one can easily catch a cold. It is a good training for the nerves to expose the body to the cold air outside immediately after waking up in the morning. It is also important not to put on too many clothes for the same reason. Massaging with a wet towel, or with a dry towel, or bathing in hot and cold bath in turn are very effective in preventing a cold. It's best to begin these training methods in the summer and continue everyday into the winter. Elderly people may massage with a dry towel every morning. This practice will promote blood circulation and keeps the skin young. Otherwise one can practise Ki exercises every morning for a quarter of an hour. It will develop the sense for temperature and perspiration, thus improving the ability to adjust the body temperature.

2. Improving the resistance of the internal organs.

The internal organs are very important for the maintenance of life. These organs are controlled by the autonomic nerves which cannot be controlled by the will of the human being. However our emotions and feelings influence the autonomic nerves. The central nerves of the autonomic nerves and those of the emotions are connected in the center of the brain. There are sympathetic nerves and parasympathetic nerves in the automatic nerves. These two act on the organs in the opposite direction. When we get angry or surprised, the sympathetic nerves are active causing a stimulated heart beat, blood vessel contraction, face pallor and stoppage or slowed movement of the stomach. The parasympathetic nerves act in the opposite direction. When the sympathetic nerves are active, the parasympathetic nerves relax and when the sympathetic nerves relax, the parasympathetic nerves are active. The activity of the parasympathetic nerves prevails when one is happy or relaxed or sleeping. During normal daytime activities the sympathetic nerves are working harder. The sympathetic nerves make one active, and the parasympathetic nerves make one rest.

The best way to improve the internal organs is to live with the activity of the parasympathetic nerves so that the cells of the internal organs accumulate energy. The internal organs work all the time without break. It is important not to waste their energy. That means the unification of mind and body is necessary for the improvement of the internal organs.

Hormones also influence the internal organs. The secretion of hormones is also controlled by the autonomic nerves. If one type of the autonomic nerves remains in constant tension, the internal organs are damaged. After a strong stimulation, one must relax.

Deep sleep is a state of unification of the mind and body and effectively recovers fatigue. Strain means the consumption of energy of the internal organs and accumulation of fatigue in the body. It shows in the blood composition. The oxygen decreases, the carbonic acid gas increases, and the waste materials are acid and make the blood also acid. This influences the maintenance of health. There are many leucocytes in the blood which are phagocytic. The phagocytosis is high when the blood is weak alkaline and as the blood becomes acid, it weakens. It is why one catches easily cold when he is tired. Decrease of oxygen in the blood due to strain causes low activity in cells of the internal organs. Evacuation of waste materials in blood is a method to increase resistance of the internal organs. Ki breathing and Ki meditation are the best ways to strengthen the internal organs. When we unify our mind and body, the mind is calm and the energy of the organic cells are not wasted and the waste materials are efficiently evacuated.

The cells are activated and there is abundant oxygen in the blood.

In addition, adequate exercise can improve the blood circulation which increases blood going to the internal organs. Exercises with the mind and body unified are even more effective.

3. Exercise

Everybody knows exercise is important to maintain health. However, many healthy people do not regularly exercise. But exercise certainly influences the human life.

a) The necessity of exercise

Modern people often take enough nourishment but work only mentally and lack physical exercise. If one lives this way over a period of time, waste materials accumulate in the body. As a result, the blood vessels become rigid and the blood pressure goes up. This is particularly dangerous when the blood vessels in the brain are involved. The lungs and heart function less so that one can exercise less, causing bad circulation. Naturally the functions of liver and kidneys decrease and one gets old. The joints get stiff, muscles and tendons become rigid, one loses the desire to exercise. Heart disease and diabetes are likely to occur. It is very important to do exercise regularly.

b) The effects of exercise

The general effects of whole body exercise are as follows:

1) The lungs efficiently gather oxygen and release carbon dioxide in the lungs. While an adult stays calm, he takes in 300 cc of oxygen per minute, while walking, 800cc, in vigorous exercise, more than 3,000 cc. The blood from the heart increases, the lactic acid which is accumulated in the body is oxidized and evacuated in the form of carbon dioxide and water. Both the lungs and the heart must work vigorously, otherwise they will become weak.

2) The blood vessels of the skin enlarge and perspiration is activated to prevent the rise of temperature. This makes the metabolism of the skin vigorous. And waste materials are released in perspiration.

3) The blood vessels are enlarged, causing them to be elastic, thus preventing high blood pressure.

4) The metabolism of brain nerves is activated. The secretion of hormones increase and the life power is enhanced.

5) The unnecessary fat accumulated in the body is burnt and evacuated. The muscle tissues increase and energy accumulates in the body.

6) The internal organs have a lot of blood vessels. They function all the time without break. The waste materials are easily accumulated and can cause senility.

Exercise prevent this and keep the internal organs young.

c) Quantity and quality of exercise

There are many sorts of exercise. It is better to choose an exercise of the whole body, which one can continue everyday without getting fatigue. For example, a weak person or elderly person can walk or do Ki exercises. A strong person or a young person can do aikido or other sports. The important thing is to continue without strain. The quantity of exercise is easily measured from outside but the quality of exercise is difficult to measure. However, the quality is more important to one's health. Unification of mind and body means the whole mind and the whole body participates in the exercise. All the internal organs, bones, muscles, and the brain are working according to their natural principles so that the original life power works at its maximum force. When doing any exercise, if one does it with four basic principles to unify mind and body, the quality of exercise is at its highest.

4. Air conditioning sickness

The human body adapts itself to the environments in order to maintain life. One can make a strong body making use of this adaptability. However if the body receives a stimulus exceeding limit of resistance, the body is shocked.

For example, there is an adaptability toward the change of temperature. When the temperature is high, the skin blood vessels enlarge, the heart gives more blood, and perspiration prevents the rise of the temperature of the body. When one goes to a place which is air conditioned with a lower temperature, the skin blood vessels contract and the decreases in body temperature is prevented. This is controlled by the autonomic nerves.

The autonomic nerves adjust the body to the environments. The nervous system can be classified into the cerebrospinal system and the autonomic nervous system. The cerebrospinal system controls the motor nerves and the autonomic nervous system controls the internal organs, endocrine system, blood vessels, etc. The autonomic nervous system is so important to the maintenance of life that it is sometimes called the system of life nerves. The autonomic nervous system consists of the sympathetic nervous system and the parasympathetic nervous system. These two systems function opposite to each other.

The central system of the autonomic nerves is influenced by the emotion. Anger, anxiety, surprise, and emergencies excite the sympathetic nerves which in turn makes the heart beat faster, the blood pressure rise, the breathing increase, the pupils of the eyes dilate, and perspiration and the secretion of saliva decrease. In this way the autonomic nervous system moves with the stimuli of the environment and the emotions so that the human body can survive, adapting itself to its environment.

A sudden change of temperature has a large influence on the mind and body. If there are several tens of change of temperature, the autonomic nervous system consumes too much energy and finally becomes exhausted. At that time the nerves become too sensitive and when there is one unit of stimulus, the nerves give ten units of stimuli to the brain. This is the sickness caused by air conditioning.

a) Symptoms

The blood vessels in the muscle contract continually so the nourishment to the muscles is low. This causes stiff shoulders, pain in the loins, fatigue of the whole body, dizziness, loss of appetite, quick heart beating, etc. Finally it could caused the muscle to cramp. The secretion of hormones is blocked and the equilibrium of the whole body is broken. The ovaries may fail to function properly which can lead to metrorrhagia. The suprarenal hormone secretion is inhibited, which causes low resistance to bacteria and recovery from colds or pneumonia becomes difficult.

b) Prevention and cure

First, it is better to live without air conditioning. If the room is air conditioned cool, first go to a relatively less cool place and try to adjust as slowly as possible. The difference between the exterior temperature and the air conditioned room should be less than five degrees centigrade.

Secondly, avoid fatigue and do not strain the nerves. When the nerves have a lot of energy, they can adjust to the change of temperature. The best prevention and cure is Ki breathing. Ki breathing makes the mind and body strong and gives energy to the nerves. By doing Ki breathing one perspires, the blood vessels enlarge, and one can correct an abnormal condition. Try Ki breathing 30 minutes to one hour every day. Besides that, if you can, exercise so that you perspire well and then take a bath. The muscles will get softer and the mind will become more stable.

Chapter $\boxed{4}$ Psychosomatic Medicine

1. What is psychosomatic medicine?

   Psychosomatic medicine has been known since the presentation of the stress theory. Stress is the reaction of the body to the change of mind which is caused by fear, anxiety, temperature change, injury, etc. Of course, medicine which concerns the human being and disease cannot work with the idea of separation of mind and body. One cannot treat a disease with only the mind or the body. All the best doctors have the attitude to look at the whole human being when they treat a patient. However as modern medicine developed scientifically and technologically, some doctors started to look only the physical symptoms and forget the mind. Because of this tendency of modern medicine, false religions and charm cures have become popular. As a result of the stress theory, science can now measure the physical change caused by the mental change. Now science is obliged to think mind and body together. The change of mind influences the body and sometimes cause disease. Or physical change causes mental change and sometimes results in neurosis. Naturally nearly all the diseases can be called psychosomatic. However, so called psychosomatic medicine treats only the desease in which the mental aspect plays a big role. The following are examples:

   (1) The mental attitude causes the disease to worsen.

   (2) The mental changes starts the disease.

   (3) Neurosis

2. What is the mind?

   The nature of the mind is movement. It never stops. This is something one should not forget when one wants to control the mind. Master Tohei explains this as the difference between living calmness and the dead calmness. Knowing this difference is very important to understand the mind. The mind can be classified as the material mind, plant mind, animal mind (or instinctive mind), human mind, and the universal mind. The material mind is the property of matter. For example hydrogen atom consists of one atomic nucleus and one electron, which is moving around the nucleus in a high speed. This state forms the atom. The property of the hydrogen atom is called the mind of the hydrogen atom. When this property vanishes, the hydrogen atom can no longer exist. The plant mind is the property of a plant. It includes reproduction, growth, breathing, circulation, etc. The animal mind has appetite, sexual desires, and other instincts. The human mind introduces judgement of good and bad, right and wrong, memorizing and learning and teaching. Those are characteristics of the human being. The animal mind and the human mind are abstract and invisible. These minds are performed in the brain.

The animal mind and the human mind are generally treated in psychosomatic medicine. Among the human mind there is an ability to change the mind (will power). This mind controls the mind and body and instincts. When this calm mind is one with the universe, it is called the universal mind. The mechanism of the mind is not well-known. However, if we assume the mind is a particle smaller than light, this particle of the mind must be created in the brain. As Master Tohei has mentioned, "The refined body is the mind. The gross mind is the body."

CONCLUSION

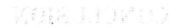

Conclusion

Modern science has enabled us to live longer than last generations, however not necessarily in a healthier way, especially when we get older. Nowadays people are too dependent on modern medicine though many problems could be solved more simply using Kiatsu and the principles of Ki.

Moreover, if one lives with mind and body unified using the principles of Ki, sickness can be avoided. Prevention is desirable to cure. Thus the Ki exercises thoroughly explained in part 2 of this book, if practised every day, will lead to a healthier life.

Dr. Arrizumi explained in part 3 of this book through an holistic approach the relation of Ki with the mind and body. It is hoped that readers will not presuppose unification of mind and body to be a mystic or purely philosophical theory. Refined body is mind and gross mind is body. Unification of mind and body is a human being's original and natural state. Therefore it is my sincere hope that as many as possible will learn to unify their minds and bodies. In this way the infinite powers of the universe can be used to help others.

The Kiatsu Ryoho Gakuin (Kiatsu Therapy School) was established in April of 1980 in Tokyo at the Ki No Kenkyukai H.Q.

This two years' program consists of a series of lectures and practical training of Kiatsu Techniques and unification of mind and body exercises. Classes are offered in the morning and the evening and students are welcomed to attend either session. Students are to attend class three times per week. Each class is three hours. The first semester is from April to the middle of July and the second semister is from September to the middle of February. After two years of study a student can be certified as a Kiatsu Therapist.

Students from overseas are welcome with the condition that he understands English.
The entrance examination is held in February every year.

KI NO KENKYUKAI H.Q.

101 USHIGOME HEIM, 2-30 HARAMACHI, SHINJUKU-KU, TOKYO
 Tel. 03-353-3461, 3462

Branches of KI NO KENKYUKAI

Hawaii Ki Society Federation
620 Waipa Lane, Honolulu, HI 96817, U.S.A;   Tel: 808-845-3064

Eastcoast Ki Society Federation
c/o Shizuo Imaizumi
201 East 19th St. Apt. #14J, New York, NY 10003,
U.S.A.   Tel: 212-673-7418

Northwest Ki Society Federation
P.O.Box 02025, Portland, OR 97202, U.S.A.   Tel: 503-223-9124

Midland Ki Society Federation
P.O.Box 818, Boulder, CO 80306, U.S.A.   Tel: 303-442-0505

Northern California Ki Society Federation
1235 De Haro St., San Francisco, CA 94107, U.S.A. Tel: 415-647-8157

Ki No Kenkyukai Italia
Costa de Magnoli 29, 50125 Firenze, Italia   Tel: 055-211962

Ki Federation of Great Britain
c/o Kenneth Williams
Isle Port House , 4 Isle Port Road, Highbridge
Somerset, England

Ki No Kenkyukai Bruxelles
70 Rue Lieutenant Liedel, Bruxelles,   Tel: 02-523-0621
1070, Belgium

Ki-Aikido Dojo Berlin
Hedemannstr. 11, 1000 Berlin 61, West Germany   Tel: 030-251-4696

New Zealand Ki Society
P.O.Box 1140 Auckland, New Zealand